Complete Pathology
for Complementary Therapies

Written in partnership with the Association of Reflexologists

Essential Training Solutions Ltd.
PO Box 5116
Badby
Daventry
Northants
NN11 3ZB

+44(0)1604 879110
www.essential-training.co.uk

ISBN: 978-0-9553425-7-8

Disclaimer

Every effort has been made to ensure that the information and advice given in this book is accurate and up to date. Whilst the information and advice given throughout is believed to be true, safe and accurate at the time of production, Essential Training Solutions Ltd and the Association of Reflexologists cannot accept any legal responsibility or liability for any errors or omissions that may be made. Essential Training Solutions Ltd and the Association of Reflexologists accept no legal responsibility or liability whatsoever for the accuracy of the information, conclusions that may be drawn from it, how the information is interpreted and implemented by the reader or any third party, and any injury, howsoever caused, to any person. This is the basis on which the information is presented.

Contents

This page has been intentionally left blank.

<u>Acne</u>

Definition: Chronic skin disease affecting practically all adolescents.

Possible Causes: Over-activity of the sebaceous glands, which produce the oily secretion called sebum. The excess sebum secreted causes the hair follicle to block. These glands are sensitive to hormone levels and so puberty is often a common time for the disease to be triggered. In women the menstrual cycle and pregnancy can also be triggers. Stress worsens the condition, as sufferers tend to pick their spots more when under pressure. There is often a presence of micro-organisms.

General Signs and Symptoms: Sebaceous glands become blocked and infected. This leads to small spots or lumps commonly on the face, back and chest. The face is usually affected most due to the greater number of sebaceous glands.

Conventional Medical Treatment: Mild acne can be treated topically with creams and gels. In more severe cases antibiotics are used too. In extreme instances a medication called isotretinoin can be prescribed by only a dermatologist because it can cause serious side effects and must be carefully monitored.

Prognosis: Most will have repeated episodes for several years and then the acne usually disappears. Treatments tend to be effective, taking about 2-3 months to work. Severe cases may leave scarring but prompt treatment can help to reduce this.

Holistic Advice: Requires a good skin hygiene routine using non-greasy, unfragranced, cleansing products. Wash hands before touching the face to reduce the spread of bacteria, and eat a balanced diet.

Addison's Disease

Definition: Disorder of the adrenal glands. Also known as primary adrenal insufficiency or hypoadrenalism.

Possible Causes: The result of the failure of the adrenal cortex to produce normal quantities of the steroid hormones cortisol and aldosterone. The most common reason is an autoimmune condition, in which the body creates antibodies that attack the adrenal cortex. If 90% of the cortex is destroyed, the adrenals are unable to produce sufficient hormones, so inducing the symptoms. Genetic composition may predispose some to autoimmune Addison's disease. Other conditions such as tuberculosis, HIV infection, some fungal infections (e.g. ringworm), genetic defect and cancer may also destroy the function of the adrenals. On occasions the adrenals may have to be removed altogether. Vitiligo, type 1 diabetes and hypothyroidism have also been linked to Addison's.

General Signs and Symptoms: Symptoms develop slowly and begin with tiredness, vague feeling of ill health, lack of energy, muscle weakness, dehydration, increased thirst, low blood pressure, increased need to urinate and a loss of appetite but a craving for salty foods. Any situation that increases the stress levels makes the symptoms worse. As the disorder progresses, or if the body is under additional stress, the initial symptoms worsen and may be accompanied by falling blood pressure on standing, dizziness, fainting, nausea, vomiting, diarrhoea, abdominal, joint or back pain, muscle cramps, exhaustion, depression and a brownish discoloration of the skin (particularly on the palms, scars, elbows, knuckles and knees). If the symptoms above are very severe it could be indicative of an adrenal crisis. This is a medical emergency and can be fatal. Although a rare condition, it is twice as common in women than men.

Conventional Medical Treatment: Corticosteroid replacement therapy is used to replace the missing hormones. This is usually taken orally but can be administered by injection. When the underlying cause is another condition, treating that will obviously treat the Addison's.

Prognosis: For autoimmune Addison's medication is permanently required, but when the condition is appropriately treated neither quality nor quantity of life should be affected. Left untreated the disease can lead to an adrenal crisis which can be fatal.

Holistic Advice: Wear a medical alert bracelet to inform medical personnel in case of an accident. Try to keep balanced and manage stress levels. Join an Addison's disease support group.

Alopecia

Definition: Loss of hair and sometimes baldness.

Possible Causes: Sudden and generally temporary significant hair loss is thought to be caused by immune system problems, anaemia, infection, stress, shock or food allergies. May occur following an illness or side effect of drugs, particularly cancer drugs. May be a sign of thyroid problems. Male-pattern baldness (see below) is caused by oversensitive hair follicles.

General Signs and Symptoms: The commonest form of hair loss is androgenic alopecia, or male-pattern baldness (although it can affect women too). The balding process is gradual, usually starting with a receding hairline. Alopecia areata involves the sudden and generally temporary loss of patches of hair and mostly affects teenagers and young adults. When the hair grows back it is fine and white before regaining its original colour. If all the hair on the scalp is lost, the condition is called alopecia totalis. If all body hair is lost, it is called alopecia universalis. Telogen effluvium is a common type of alopecia in which there is a widespread thinning of the hair, rather than the presence of bald patches.

Conventional Medical Treatment: There are drugs that can be effective to some degree in treating male-pattern baldness, but there is no really effective treatment for alopecia areata. The use of steroids may help prevent hair loss and promote hair re-growth but the condition often returns when the treatment ends and there can be side effects. For extensive or total hair loss, immunotherapy, dithranol cream and UV light treatment can be used but they all carry possible serious side effects.

Prognosis: In most cases of alopecia areata the hair grows back after about a year.

Holistic Advice: Consider the whole person and identify the cause of any stress. Baldness itself can lead to stress, so the emotional needs of the person are paramount. A flattering haircut may also make a difference, and tattooing and the use of wigs can help to alleviate the obvious signs of this condition.

Alzheimer's Disease

Definition: A progressive deterioration in mental ability due to degeneration of brain tissue. It is the most common cause of dementia (the progressive loss of mental abilities).

Possible Causes: Brain cells degenerate, causing a build up of an abnormal protein that worsens the condition by destroying more brain cells. This shrinkage of the brain results in dementia. The protein also affects the brain's ability to transmit nerve impulses. The exact cause is unknown but risk factors include age, family history, Down's syndrome, having suffered whiplash or head injury and (possibly) the level of aluminium in the body.

General Signs and Symptoms: The symptoms vary from one person to another and the speed of onset can vary too. Generally the symptoms go through 3 stages, mild, moderate and severe. Early mild symptoms may include forgetfulness, poor concentration, confusion, difficulty saying the right words, difficulty understanding written or spoken language, and wandering and getting lost even in familiar surroundings. At this stage the sufferer is aware of the symptoms and this can lead to depression and anxiety. As the condition progresses there may be mood swings, obsessive or repetitive behaviour, personality changes, sleep problems, slow movements, unsteadiness, hallucinations and delusions. The body becomes more physically affected as the condition progresses with incontinence, difficulty swallowing, difficulty changing position and weight loss, and there is an increased risk of infection. The short term and long term memory may be completely lost. It is likely that those in the severe stage of the disease will require full time care.

Conventional Medical Treatment: The stage of the condition will be assessed with tests such as the mini mental state examination (MMSE). Various drugs (e.g. donepezil) can be prescribed to slow the loss of mental function. Some of the symptoms of the condition such as depression and sleeping problems may be relieved by antidepressants. A care plan will be drawn up to support day-to-day needs.

Prognosis: There is no cure, but treatment can slow the progression of the disease.

Holistic Advice: Brain function can be helped by not smoking or drinking large quantities of alcohol, taking regular exercise, eating a balanced, healthy diet, and keeping the brain stimulated by learning new skills and participating in activities.

Amenorrhoea

Definition: Absence of menstruation. There are 2 types – primary amenorrhoea, which is a failure to start menstruation, and secondary amenorrhoea, which is the absence of menstruation in a woman who has previously been menstruating.

Possible Causes: It is obviously normal not to menstruate prior to puberty, during pregnancy and breastfeeding, after the menopause or post-hysterectomy. Also, when women stop taking the contraceptive pill it is not uncommon to have a temporary cessation of menstruation. However, at other times it may be indicative of severe weight loss, excessive exercise or an underlying disorder such as polycystic ovary syndrome, ovarian failure, thyroid or pituitary gland disorders, or eating disorders. Stress, depression, anxiety, a sudden fright or intense grief, some medications and drugs, and long-term illness may also cause hormonal disturbances that may lead to amenorrhoea.

General Signs and Symptoms: Absence of menstrual flow in women who should otherwise be having periods.

Conventional Medical Treatment: The underlying cause must be ascertained and treated. Successfully treating any underlying medical disorder will usually result in menstruation. The sufferer may be encouraged, as appropriate, to gain weight, reduce exercise and take counselling or psychological therapy. If the cause cannot be treated, hormonal treatment may be used to restart menstruation.

Prognosis: The underlying cause can usually be treated, which results in the return of menstruation.

Holistic Advice: Identifying the cause is a priority. Remember that pregnancy is contra-indicated to some complementary healthcare treatments. Try to combat stress.

Anaemia (Iron Deficiency)

Definition: Deficiency or abnormality of haemoglobin.

Possible Causes: There are several types of anaemia. Iron deficiency is by far the most common. Iron is required for the body to make haemoglobin, which stores and transports oxygen. An iron deficiency impairs the body's ability to make haemoglobin resulting in anaemia. There are many causes of iron deficiency including bleeding from the digestive tract, heavy menstrual bleeding, pregnancy, trauma resulting in blood loss, a variety of medical conditions, a lack of iron in the diet and malabsorption problems. The prolonged use of aspirin and nonsteroidal anti-inflammatory drugs can cause bleeding from the stomach lining. The causes of other types of anaemia include a lack of vitamin B12 or folic acid, inherited abnormalities of haemoglobin, the excessive rapid destruction of red blood cells and the failure to produce sufficient red blood cells.

General Signs and Symptoms: The condition may develop slowly showing symptoms such as tiredness, lethargy, weakness, shortness of breath, palpitations, headache, faintness, fading complexion, pale colour on inside of eyelids, brittle nails, cracks in the skin at the sides of the mouth, smooth tongue and an increased respiratory rate.

Conventional Medical Treatment: Establishing the underlying cause is a priority so it can be treated. The iron levels in the body can be restored using iron supplements and an iron-rich diet. The iron level should be monitored regularly. In extreme cases a blood transfusion may be necessary.

Prognosis: Establishing and treating the cause and raising the iron levels should cure the anaemia. Serious or long-term problems are rare.

Holistic Advice: Eat red meat, dried fruit and iron-rich vegetables regularly. Reduce tea and coffee intake. Seek dietary advice.

Angina

Definition: A syndrome caused by a restriction of the blood supply to the heart. There are 2 types, stable and unstable. In stable angina the symptoms are brought on by exercise, subside at rest, and usually develop gradually over time. In unstable angina the symptoms develop rapidly and can persist at rest.

Possible Causes: Angina is indicative of an inadequate blood supply to the heart muscle. Stable angina is commonly due to coronary heart disease in which the coronary arteries harden and narrow (atherosclerosis), reducing their ability to supply blood. At rest the supply may be sufficient, but during exercise or stress the heart may receive an insufficient supply of blood which triggers the syndrome. Unstable angina can be caused by the rupture of the fatty deposits in the arteries which then interfere with the blood flow causing blood clots. The blood clots can quickly grow, reducing the blood supply to the heart. Risk factors for angina include a high fat diet, a high cholesterol level, smoking, hypertension, diabetes, age, obesity, high alcohol consumption and family history. Less commonly angina can be caused by a temporary spasm of the coronary arteries, damaged heart valves and anaemia.

General Signs and Symptoms: An attack of stable angina is typified by pain or discomfort in the chest, often radiating to the neck, jaw and down the left arm. There may be sweating, breathlessness, belching and nausea. It is usually triggered by exercise but can be aggravated by exposure to cold or immediately after eating a meal. The symptoms subside during rest. The symptoms of unstable angina are the same, but they can develop without the usual triggers, last for longer, and can persist at rest. Attacks of unstable angina may not respond to the usual treatment and should be treated as a medical emergency.

Conventional Medical Treatment: For stable angina a wide range of medication is used to relieve symptoms during an attack (e.g. glycerol trinitrate spray or tablets), help prevent further attacks (e.g. beta blockers) and reduce the chance of a heart attack or stroke (e.g. statins). Surgical techniques such as coronary angioplasty (to widen the narrowing) and artery bypass grafts (to bypass the restriction) can be used. For unstable angina the emergency treatment focuses on preventing blood clots forming using blood-thinning drugs. The medication/surgery required is then established.

Prognosis: The outlook depends on the extent of coronary heart disease and the presence of other factors such as hypertension and additional chronic conditions. Taking the correct balance of medications and making lifestyle changes can improve the prognosis. Coronary heart disease carries an increased risk of a heart attack or stroke.

Holistic Advice: Lifestyle changes are very important to prevent the condition or to prevent the condition from worsening. Stop smoking and lose any excess weight. Take regular exercise and reduce stress levels. Maintain a healthy low fat, high fibre diet. Many people with coronary heart disease live in fear of a heart attack and feel hopeless, out of control and depressed, so address these issues in any complementary healthcare treatment. Support groups can be of use. Any unexplained chest pains that a client reports to you requires you to inform them to seek medical attention.

Appendicitis

Definition: Inflammation of the appendix.

Possible Causes: The appendix becomes filled with bacteria that produce pus, causing the appendix to swell. This can be caused by infection (e.g. a stomach infection) or an obstruction (e.g. hard piece of faeces) in the appendix that causes a bacterial infection. Sometimes the cause is unknown.

General Signs and Symptoms: Sudden onset of pain in the abdomen that shifts to the lower-right and gradually gets worse over several hours. This can be accompanied by nausea, vomiting, loss of appetite, constipation or diarrhoea, and a fever. Constant, worsening abdominal pain should be considered a medical emergency.

Conventional Medical Treatment: For mild cases antibiotics may be successful in reducing the inflammation, but in most cases the appendix will have to be surgically removed.

Prognosis: If left untreated the appendix may burst which can lead to potentially fatal consequences such as blood poisoning and peritonitis (inflammation of the abdominal lining). Removing the appendix has no detrimental effect on health and wellbeing.

Holistic Advice: It is thought that a high fibre diet may reduce the incidence of appendicitis.

Asthma

Definition: Intermittent narrowing of the airways, causing shortness of breath and wheezing.

Possible Causes: The bronchi become inflamed and narrow when they are irritated and mucus production increases. The muscles of the bronchi also contract making the airways narrower still. The irritation may be caused by sensitivity to certain substances, allergic reactions or other triggers, e.g. dust mites, animal fur, pollen, tobacco smoke, chemical fumes, atmospheric pollution, certain medicines, foods containing sulphites, stress, cold air and chest infections. It is thought that a combination of genetic, environmental and dietary factors may cause the condition. Risk factors include a family history of asthma, suffering from other allergic conditions (e.g. eczema), having bronchitis or being exposed to tobacco smoke as a child, being born prematurely and being born with a low birth weight.

General Signs and Symptoms: Difficulty breathing, breathlessness, wheezing, coughing and a tight chest. The severity of asthma attacks varies enormously from mild to life threatening. Symptoms such as an increase in pulse rate, more wheezing, and a feeling of agitation or restlessness, can indicate that the attack is worsening. In a severe attack, breathing may become very difficult, causing the lips and finger nails to turn blue, the nostrils to flare and pulse race. A severe attack should be treated as a medical emergency.

Conventional Medical Treatment: The aim is to eliminate symptoms and reduce the severity and frequency of future attacks. Medicines are usually administered using an inhaler. Bronchodilators are used to help alleviate the symptoms, and corticosteroids can be given to help prevent another attack. Lifestyle changes and diet play an important role.

Prognosis: The narrowing of the airways is usually reversible, either occurring naturally or with the use of medicines. However, in some chronic cases the inflammation may lead to an irreversible obstruction of the airways. Asthma can lead to serious respiratory complications and can be fatal.

Holistic Advice: Stop smoking. Maintain a healthy weight, keep to a healthy diet and exercise regularly. Yoga and gentle exercise can help keep the whole body in balance, thus helping it to cope with asthma and its associated anxiety. Practitioners should be fully trained to deal with asthmatic attacks before treating patients with asthma. During an attack, always remain calm and reassure the person. Seek medical advice if the condition worsens or persists.

Atherosclerosis

Definition: A progressive condition in which the medium and large arteries become clogged by cholesterol and fatty substances. It is a type of arteriosclerosis and can attribute to cardiovascular diseases such as heart attacks, strokes, coronary heart disease and peripheral artery disease.

Possible Causes: Arteries naturally begin to harden and narrow with age but the process can be accelerated by high fat diets and high "bad" cholesterol (low density lipoprotein) levels. The cholesterol sticks to the wall of the arteries and the fatty deposits build up over time. Platelets may worsen the condition by collecting on the fatty deposits forming blood clots. Risk factors include smoking, lack of exercise, hypertension, being overweight, diabetes, high alcohol intake, family history, ethnicity and air pollution.

General Signs and Symptoms: Symptoms do not usually arise until the blood flow becomes restricted or blocked and then the symptoms depend on the location of the arteries affected. For example, if the atherosclerosis is in the arteries of the legs, causing peripheral artery disease, cramping pains and numbness will be felt in the lower limbs. Angina is brought on by atherosclerosis of the coronary arteries and the narrowing of these arteries can lead to a heart attack. Blood clots can form as a result of atherosclerosis and cause heart attacks (if in the coronary arteries) and strokes (if blood supply to the brain is restricted). Atherosclerosis can also weaken the artery walls causing bulges called aneurysms. If the aneurysm ruptures the blood loss can prove fatal.

Conventional Medical Treatment: The treatment focuses on preventing the condition from getting worse and triggering cardiovascular disease. Drugs can be used to lessen the risk factors by lowering cholesterol levels (e.g. statins), lowering blood pressure (e.g. ACE inhibitors), and preventing blood clots (e.g. anti-platelets and aspirin). Surgery may be possible to widen the affected artery or bypass the restriction.

Prognosis: Lifestyle changes and medication can slow the progress. Left untreated the outlook is poor and it is a major cause of a heart attack, stroke and poor peripheral circulation.

Holistic Advice: Lifestyle changes are very important to prevent the condition or to prevent the condition from worsening. Stop smoking and lose any excess weight. Take regular exercise and reduce stress levels. Maintain a healthy low fat, high fibre diet.

Athlete's Foot

Definition: Fungal disease of the skin on the feet, commonly between the toes.

Possible Causes: Fungal infection caused by the fungus dermatophyte, yeasts and moulds, often picked up in warm places with humid environments such as swimming pools and changing rooms. Can also be caused by the constant sweating of the feet which causes the bacteria on the feet to multiply and infect the skin. It is contagious and so care must be taken to avoid direct or indirect contact.

General Signs and Symptoms: In the area of the infection the skin tends to be inflamed, moist, flaky, itchy and painful. Sometimes it has small blisters or a rash. In severe cases, toenails can be affected and may crumble and separate from the nail bed.

Conventional Medical Treatment: Antifungal creams, sprays and liquids applied topically will usually quickly clear up the infection. In severe cases, a GP may prescribe oral antifungal drugs.

Prognosis: If treated effectively, the infection will usually clear up in a few days or weeks. Untreated it can last for several months, even years.

Holistic Advice: Wash feet regularly, ensuring they are dried properly – particularly between the toes. Foot powder preparations can be bought without prescription to help the feet dry out. Change socks everyday! Cotton socks are best. Avoid sharing towels to help prevent any infection from spreading.

Bell's Palsy

Definition: Weakness or paralysis of the muscles on one side of the face. The eyelid may also be affected.

Possible Causes: Damage to the facial nerve as a result of inflammation, compression or a direct wound. Victims of apoplexy (stroke) may also show symptoms of Bell's palsy. Facial palsy, of which Bell's palsy is one type, may be associated with shingles (a viral infection) and Lyme disease (a bacterial infection carried by ticks).

General Signs and Symptoms: Weakness or paralysis on one side of the face, difficulty in closing the eye, and the drooping of one side of mouth which causes drooling and speech impairment. The eye may become dry, due to the eyelid being unable to close. Pain may be experienced underneath the ear and the sense of taste may be affected. The symptoms tend to develop quickly.

Conventional Medical Treatment: Steroids to reduce the inflammation. The eye on the affected side must also be cared for to ensure it is kept clean and moist. Eye drops and ointments are commonly prescribed for this.

Prognosis: Most show an improvement within 3 weeks and 85% make a full recovery within 9 months. Long lasting nerve damage is possible but rare.

Holistic Advice: Gentle massage concentrating on the back of the head and neck may help. Consult a qualified massage practitioner. Acupressure or acupuncture may be useful in the initial stages.

Bladder Stones

Definition: Small deposits of minerals that form in the bladder.

Possible Causes: If urine remains in the bladder for too long, waste products in the urine can crystallize and form stones. Bladder stones are therefore often caused by conditions in which the ability of the bladder to fully empty is compromised, e.g. recurrent bladder infections, prostatitis, and neurological problems that affect bladder control. Other risk factors include a diet high in fat, sugar or salt, prolonged dehydration, metabolic conditions such as gout (due to the increased levels of waste products in the urine), and vitamin A or B deficiency.

General Signs and Symptoms: Some bladder stones can be passed from the bladder unnoticed. Usually, however, symptoms are experienced because the stones can irritate the wall of the bladder or block the flow of urine. Symptoms include pain when urinating, blood in the urine, lower abdominal pain, difficulty beginning to urinate, stop-start urination, the need to urinate frequently and the need to urinate in the night. Bladder stones are more common in men than women, and are more common over the age of 45.

Conventional Medical Treatment: Small stones may be flushed out by drinking more water. It may be possible to break larger stones down using lithotripsy, which involves sending high-energy shock waves through the stone to break it up so the pieces can then be flushed out. Alternatively, stones can be surgically removed.

Prognosis: Treatment to remove the stones is usually successful, but if the underlying cause remains they may recur.

Holistic Advice: Drink plenty of water. Eat a low fat, high fibre diet with plenty of fresh fruit and vegetables. Limit sugar and salt intake.

Boils

Definition: A red, painful, pus-filled swelling of the skin. A cluster of boils is referred to as a carbuncle.

Possible Causes: Bacterial infection (usually Staphylococcus aureus) of the hair follicle or sebaceous gland. As the infection spreads pus collects in the surrounding tissues. Most common in those with a low resistance to infection such as diabetics or those with HIV.

General Signs and Symptoms: Small, red, tender lump that feels warm to the touch and throbs. The tissues around the boil swell as pus accumulates. Eventually the boil forms a yellow or white head. Boils are commonly located on the neck or face, in moist areas of the body such as the armpits, and in areas subjected to friction from clothing. They are most common in teenagers and young adults.

Conventional Medical Treatment: Antibiotics may be needed if the infection looks to be spreading to the deeper layers of the skin. Doctors may drain the pus if necessary. Large boils may need to be lanced. Painkillers may be required to treat the pain.

Prognosis: Most heal without treatment within a couple of weeks. They may burst and release the pus or gradually subside. Recurrent boils may be indicative of an underlying medical condition. Secondary infections, most commonly cellulitis, are a risk if the infection spreads.

Holistic Advice: Do not squeeze the boil. The healing process may be improved by applying a cloth, made hot by soaking in warm water, to the boil for 10 minutes, 3-4 times a day. Wash your hands after touching the boil. Try to improve the immune system.

Breast Lump

Definition: A mass or swelling that can be felt in the breast tissue.

Possible Causes: Generalised lumpiness is often associated with hormonal changes at puberty, pregnancy and menstruation due to the oversensitivity of the breast tissue to female sex hormones. Mastitis (inflammation of the breast tissue) can cause breast lumps. One of the most common causes of breast lumps in pre-menopausal women is fibroadenosis. This is caused by the formation of excessive fibrous connective tissue that causes breast pain, breast enlargement and general lumpiness of the breast. One type of non-malignant breast tumour is fibroadenoma. These tumours (solid masses) can be felt as hard rubbery lumps and may be caused by an overgrowth of fibrous and glandular tissue. Fibroadenoma is most common in women in their 20s. Breast cysts (fluid filled sac in the breast tissue) can be felt as lumps too. Occasionally the breast lump may be due to an infection that has caused the development of an abscess. Lumps may also be caused by injury and fatty growths. A breast lump can also be symptomatic of breast cancer, although 9 out of 10 breast lumps are benign.

General Signs and Symptoms: Generalised lumpiness in the breast tissue or a separate, individual lump felt either deep in the breast tissue or just under the skin. There may be breast pain. The skin may dimple and the lump may cause inversion of the nipple and a bloody nipple discharge. Specific signs and symptoms vary according to the cause.

Conventional Medical Treatment: Generalised lumpiness tends to decrease after the menopause. Drugs can be given to help reduce breast pain. Small fibroadenomas do not usually need treatment and tend to become smaller or disappear within a couple of years. Larger fibroadenomas may need to be removed surgically or by laser. Breast cysts and abscesses can be drained. A variety of treatments is available for breast cancer, including lumpectomy, mastectomy, radiotherapy, chemotherapy and other drug treatments such as tamoxifen.

Prognosis: Benign breast lumps are harmless and most do not need treatment. Lumps due to breast cancer are serious. Early diagnosis significantly affects the outcome. If diagnosed before the cancer has spread to other body organs then the treatment is more likely to be successful.

Holistic Advice: Check the breasts regularly for any lumps. Any changes in the breast should be reported to a Doctor. Reduce caffeine intake and cut down on fatty foods. Wear a good supporting bra.

Bronchitis

Definition: Inflammation of the mucous membrane within the bronchial tubes.

Possible Causes: Acute bronchitis is caused by a bacterial or, more commonly, a viral infection, often developing after a cold, sore throat or flu. Smokers, those with other pulmonary (lung) diseases, and those exposed to substances that can irritate the lungs are at greater risk. In such cases the condition may become chronic.

General Signs and Symptoms: The symptoms will vary according to the severity of the attack and the extent of the inflammation. At first the symptoms of acute bronchitis can be similar to those of a common cold (e.g. sore throat, headache, blocked nose, aches and pains and a slight fever). The main symptom is a cough that may remain long after the other symptoms have gone. The cough is usually short, dry and painful at first, with fast wheezes of respiration. The chest becomes painful and tight and, as the disease progresses, the cough may become productive.

Conventional Medical Treatment: Painkillers (such as paracetamol) can be used to reduce any temperature and help with the aches. Should a secondary infection arise (usually indicated by coughing up discoloured sputum), antibiotics may be prescribed. Antibiotics are not commonly prescribed for acute bronchitis because it is usually caused by a viral infection and so they would serve no purpose.

Prognosis: Acute bronchitis is usually mild and clears up by itself. There is no cure for chronic bronchitis but lifestyle changes may help.

Holistic Advice: During an attack drink plenty of water and rest. Give up smoking and avoid smoky areas. Take advice on breathing exercises.

Bunions

Definition: A bony swelling at the base of the big toe. Called hallux valgus.

Possible Causes: Exact cause is not known but bunions may be familial. Badly fitting shoes may also be a contributing factor. They can be caused or worsened by arthritis.

General Signs and Symptoms: Big toe bends towards the middle of the foot and the second toe creating a swollen, red, bony lump on the medial edge of the foot where the first and second metatarsals are pushed apart. The skin over the bump can become thick, rough and may break. There may be pain on walking, particularly if wearing tight footwear or high heels. Bunions are more common in women than men (probably because of the high-heeled shoes!).

Conventional Medical Treatment: Treatment is only necessary if the bunion is causing pain, which may be controlled simply by wearing flat, wide shoes. Painkillers can be taken, and bunion pads and ice packs may be effective. However, bunions will only worsen over time and the only cure for them is corrective surgery.

Prognosis: Surgery is generally successful in straightening the joint and relieving the pain. However, as with all surgery, there is the chance that complications will arise. Bunion surgery can cause stiffness in the joint, pain under the ball of the foot, nerve damage and infection. There is also no guarantee that the bunion will not reform.

Holistic Advice: Wear shoes that fit – preferably wide enough to allow the toes space to move.

Bursitis

Definition: Inflammation of a bursa. Bursae are fluid-filled sacs that act as cushions between surfaces that rub together such as bones, muscles, joints and tendons, reducing friction between them.

Possible Causes: Bursae can become inflamed by injury most often as a result of repetitive action. Occasionally the inflammation may be due to infection, but this only tends to occur in those with a weakened immune system. Bursitis can also be symptomatic of joint conditions such as rheumatoid arthritis and gout. Risk factors include any activity that involves repetitive movement (e.g. joggers' ankles are at risk, as are the knees of those who regularly kneel, such as gardeners and carpet fitters) and factors that weaken the immune system, such as diabetes, HIV/AIDS, cancer treatments and heavy alcohol consumption.

General Signs and Symptoms: Pain and swelling in the affected area. This is commonly a joint such as the shoulder, elbow, knee (called housemaid's knee), ankle and hip, but may also occur on the thighs (through stretching) and buttocks (from sitting on hard surfaces). Joints may become difficult to move due to the inflammation.

Conventional Medical Treatment: Symptoms are often mild and require no treatment. Rest and taking painkillers (such as ibuprofen) will usually help the episode to pass. Protecting the area from further damage and using ice packs and compression can help. Elevating the affected area (if possible) may also help the inflammation.

Prognosis: Symptoms usually pass in a couple of weeks.

Holistic Advice: Protect joints that are at risk (e.g. use knee pads if often kneeling). Take regular breaks from repetitive actions and warm up adequately before exercise. Boost the immune system. Maintaining muscle strength and tone will help protect joints.

Cancer

Definition: Term used to describe malignant disease. There are many types of cancer, usually named after the area of the body affected – e.g. breast cancer, lung cancer, prostate cancer, pancreatic cancer. The disease may then spread through the blood and lymphatic systems. There are many different terms used to describe the type of cancer such as malignant tumours (a solid mass of cells), carcinoma (malignant epithelial tumour), sarcoma (malignant tumour of the connective tissue), malignant melanoma (cancer affecting the pigment cells in the skin that can spread to other parts of the body), lymphoma (cancer of the lymphatic system), and leukaemia (cancer of bone marrow in which the white blood cells multiply uncontrollably).

Possible Causes: A cell may become cancerous when certain genes that control vital processes such as cell division become damaged. These faulty genes may be inherited or caused by carcinogens (cancer-causing agents) such as tobacco smoke and sunlight. Most cancers appear to be triggered by several factors, inherited and environmental. Key environmental factors also include diet, environmental pollution, alcohol, viral infections, age and hormonal influences. There may be psychological factors involved too. Depression, grief and severe mental stresses may affect vulnerability.

General Signs and Symptoms: The body's cells begin to grow and reproduce in an uncontrollable way. These cancer cells invade healthy tissue and destroy it. The majority of cancers produce a solid tumour in a specific part of the body. The signs and symptoms vary according to the location of the tumour e.g. cancer of the stomach may cause dyspepsia; cancer of the bowel may produce diarrhoea or constipation; lymphoma may cause persistent and painless swellings in the neck, armpits, or groin caused by enlarged lymph glands. Skin cancers may be seen as hard swellings on the skin's surface that may break down and ulcerate.

Conventional Medical Treatment: The treatment is determined by the type of cancer and its severity.

Prognosis: Varies from type to type. Early diagnosis is very important.

Holistic Advice: Eating a healthy diet, taking regular exercise and not smoking may all contribute to preventing cancer.

<u>Carpal Tunnel Syndrome</u>

Definition: Nerve compression at the wrist.

Possible Causes: Pressure on the median nerve as it passes through the carpal tunnel. The carpal tunnel is a small tunnel that runs from the bottom of the wrist to the lower palm through which several tendons pass, as well as the median nerve. The median nerve has both sensory and motor functions so it affects not only how the hand feels but how it moves. Carpal tunnel syndrome may be familial, and certain conditions such as gout, lupus, hypothyroidism, diabetes, pregnancy, obesity, rheumatoid arthritis, oedema and lyme disease may increase its risk of developing. Keeping the hand or wrist in one position or carrying out repetitive tasks may trigger or worsen the condition. Structural abnormalities of the wrist may also cause this syndrome.

General Signs and Symptoms: Tingling, numbness or pain in the median nerve, which affects the thumb, index finger, middle finger and half of the ring finger. Pain may be worse at night. Manually dexterity may be reduced. Moving the hand or shaking the wrist can help to alleviate the symptoms.

Conventional Medical Treatment: Symptoms may clear up without treatment. Wrist splints and corticosteroid injections can be used and, in severe cases surgery may be required to reduce the pressure on the nerve. When the condition is brought on by an underlying condition, treating that condition may help the carpal tunnel syndrome.

Prognosis: Left untreated it can lead to permanent nerve damage.

Holistic Advice: Avoid over-straining neck, arms and hands. Do not lift heavy objects. Seek regular massage to the neck and shoulders. Relax with head and neck well supported on a regular basis. Review seating position during driving and computer work. Deal with any obesity. Chiropractic may be of benefit.

Chilblains

Definition: Small, itchy, painful, red-purple swellings on the fingers, toes and other extremities such as the ears and nose.

Possible Causes: Excessive narrowing of blood vessels under the skin in cold weather then, as the vessels dilate when the body warms, the sudden increased blood flow causes blood to leak into the tissues. Chilblains may be acute, healing a couple of weeks after exposure to the cold, or chronic, causing persistent problems. Risk factors include poor circulation, lupus, family history, poor diet, and exposure to cold and damp environments, Raynaud's disease and smoking.

General Signs and Symptoms: Typically occur a couple of hours after exposure to the cold. The chilblains are painful when exposed to the cold and become very itchy and produce a burning sensation as the skin warms up again. The affected area may become red and swollen and in extreme cases the skin may break forming sores and blisters. Children and the elderly are most susceptible.

Conventional Medical Treatment: If the chilblains become infected antibiotics may be prescribed. Otherwise an over the counter mixture of friar's balsam and iodine can be painted on the site, lanolin ointment can be used to keep the skin supple, and antiseptic cream can help to avoid infection.

Prognosis: Chilblains do not usually cause permanent damage and will normally disappear without treatment if the affected area is protected from the cold, but they may recur. In extreme cases they may lead to infection, skin discoloration, ulcers and scarring.

Holistic Advice: Keep warm! Dress appropriately in the winter and avoid drafts. Take regular exercise to promote circulation. Stop smoking and avoid tight clothing and shoes that may restrict circulation. Don't try to reheat up the hands or feet quickly when they get cold by putting them on a heater etc because this will speed up the sudden return of the blood and worsen the pain and the condition.

Cirrhosis

Definition: Irreversible scarring of the liver.

Possible Causes: Healthy liver tissue is destroyed and replaced by scar tissue which starts to block the flow of blood through the liver so reducing liver function. This is usually caused by excessive alcohol consumption or the hepatitis C virus. Less common causes include hepatitis B, inherited liver disease, non-alcoholic steatohepatitis and autoimmune hepatitis. The first stage of alcoholic liver disease is known as fatty liver. Fatty liver usually reverses after 3-6 months of abstinence from alcohol. If drinking is not halted, the second stage is alcoholic hepatitis (liver inflammation). Some may still recover from this stage if alcohol is given up. Cirrhosis is the third stage and is irreversible. The government safe drinking guidelines recommend that men drink no more than 21 units a week (and no more than 3-4 units a day) and women drink no more than 14 units a week (and no more than 2-3 units a day). Women drinkers are at a greater risk of developing cirrhosis, although cirrhosis affects more men than women (because more men drink heavily).

General Signs and Symptoms: The early stages of cirrhosis often pass symptom-free. However, after several years of heavy drinking the scar tissue builds up and the liver begins to lose function. The resulting symptoms include loss of appetite, weight loss, discomfort in the upper-right side of the abdomen, tiredness, nausea and very itchy skin. In later stages of cirrhosis there are many symptoms including jaundice, oedema, vomiting blood, tendency to bruise easily, rapid heartbeat, breathlessness, dark, tarry faeces and a build up of fluid in the legs and abdomen. Ultimately the liver may fail.

Conventional Medical Treatment: Cirrhosis cannot be cured so the treatment focuses on preventing it from progressing and managing the symptoms. The treatment depends on the cause. If it's due to alcohol, lifestyle changes must be made. If it's due to an underlying disease such as viral hepatitis or autoimmune hepatitis, medication can be given. The treatment given to ease the symptoms will depend on the symptoms being experienced. The only treatment for liver failure is a liver transplant.

Prognosis: The outlook depends on the severity of the liver damage. Many can live with cirrhosis for many years, but it can lead to liver cancer and liver failure.

Holistic Advice: Cirrhosis can be largely avoided by drinking within the guidelines, and taking precautions to avoid infection from the hepatitis B and C viruses.

<u>Congenital Heart Disease</u>

Definition: One or more defects of the heart that are present from birth. There are two main types – cyanotic and acyanotic. When the heart defect results in too little oxygen in the blood, it is called cyanotic heart disease. In acyanotic heart disease, there is sufficient oxygen in the blood but the defect in the heart prevents the blood from being circulated correctly.

Possible Causes: Congenital heart disease is the most common birth defect but the cause of the abnormal foetal development is largely unknown. It can sometimes run in families, indicating a genetic link. Congenital heart disease may also be associated with genetic disorders such as Down's syndrome. Exposure of the foetus to excessive alcohol and drugs may increase the risk. If the mother contracts certain infections (e.g. rubella) in early pregnancy, or is diabetic, there is an increased likelihood that the baby will be born with this condition. Septal defects (commonly called hole in the heart), in which there is a hole in the wall that divides the left and right sides of the heart, is one of the most common defects. Heart valves, the aorta and other blood vessels may be defective, and in some cases there may be multiple defects.

General Signs and Symptoms: Many defects result in a shortness of breath, breathing difficulties, difficulty in feeding, poor appetite, sweating, chest pains, slow weight gain and delayed growth. If the defect causes low oxygen levels in the blood, the tongue and lips may appear blue and it may cause fainting.

Conventional Medical Treatment: There is a variety of surgical techniques to correct the defect. About half of babies born with congenital heart disease will require immediate surgery. The remainder will probably require surgery or medication at some later point in childhood.

Prognosis: Depends on the type of heart defect and its severity. Even very severe defects can often be successfully corrected. 85% of children born with a heart defect will live to reach adulthood.

Holistic Advice: It may be possible to reduce the risk a little by the mother taking good care of herself during pregnancy.

Constipation

Definition: The infrequent, difficult or incomplete emptying of the bowel which leads to hard faeces.

Possible Causes: Can be caused by a number (and often a combination) of factors including insufficient fibre and fluids in the diet, changes in routine and eating habits, lack of exercise and immobility, anxiety and depression, and ignoring the urge to defaecate. Drinking too much alcohol and caffeine is dehydrating which makes the faeces harder and more difficult to pass. Can also be caused by some medications (e.g. antacids, antidepressants and diuretics) and is common in pregnancy. It can be symptomatic of an underlying medical condition such as colon or rectal cancer, diabetes, hypothyroidism, some nervous system disorders and irritable bowel syndrome.

General Signs and Symptoms: Less frequent or more difficult defaecation of dry, hard and lumpy faeces. Constipation can also cause stomach aches and cramps, bloating, nausea and loss of appetite.

Conventional Medical Treatment: Lifestyle changes in diet, exercise and routine may enable the condition to be relieved without the use of medication. Laxatives can be given to promote defaecation. For more serious cases suppositories and enemas may be required. Treatment is usually effective but it may take several months to re-establish regular bowel movements. Any underlying condition needs to be identified and treated appropriately.

Prognosis: Many will only experience constipation for a short time, with no impact on health. Cases of chronic constipation can cause significant pain and discomfort. It can lead to hard faeces remaining in the rectum, and liquid faeces leaking around it causing diarrhoea.

Holistic Advice: Drink plenty of water and eat a healthy, low fat but high fibre diet. Try to adopt a routine of opening the bowel at the same time every day and try not to resist the urge to defaecate. Take regular exercise and reduce stress to help the functioning of the digestive system.

Contact Dermatitis / Eczema

Definition: A condition that causes inflammation of the skin (derma- = skin, -itis = inflammation). Eczema is also known as dermatitis, although we often (incorrectly) only tend to associate eczema with atopic dermatitis, which is the most common and hereditary form of eczema and mainly affects children. Atopic dermatitis is linked to other conditions such as asthma and hay fever. We'll concentrate on contact dermatitis here. Remember it is still a type of eczema.

Possible Causes: Can be caused by allergies or irritants. Allergic contact dermatitis is caused by exposure to a substance that causes an abnormal reaction from the immune system (e.g. cosmetics, some plants, metals such as nickel or cobalt in jewellery). Irritant contact dermatitis is caused by contact to a substance that damages the skin (e.g. chemicals, detergents, perfumes, dust). Irritants are the most common cause. Stress and poor diet may play a part.

General Signs and Symptoms: Inflammation, itching, redness, dryness, cracking, blistering, scaling and weeping of the skin, crusts and secondary skin infections. Most common on the hands and face.

Conventional Medical Treatment: The best treatment is to try to avoid the allergen or irritant. Emollients, creams, lotions and ointments can be used to soften and soothe skin. In more severe cases corticosteroids may be prescribed for topical application. Any secondary infection can be treated with antibiotics. If the dermatitis fails to respond to the treatments mentioned above, a dermatologist can prescribe alitretinoin tablets. They can be prescribed only by a dermatologist because they can cause serious side effects and must be carefully monitored.

Prognosis: Dermatitis can usually be successfully managed but in some cases can have a severe and long lasting affect on quality of both personal and working life.

Holistic Advice: Ensure a good balanced diet of fresh fruit and vegetables. Drinking plenty of water can help to keep the skin hydrated. Hypoallergenic moisturisers may be of benefit. Try to avoid exposure to potential allergens and irritants. If exposure occurs, wash the affected skin as soon as possible. If exposed to irritants at work ensure employer is informed of condition and any personal protective clothing provided is used.

<u>Corns and Calluses</u>

Definition: Areas of hard, thickened skin on the hands or feet.

Possible Causes: Prolonged pressure or friction on a small area of skin. Badly fitting shoes is a major contributing factor to the development of corns and those with misshapen feet are particularly susceptible. Calluses can be caused by repetitive actions that produce pressure on the feet such as jogging, or an uneven distribution of body weight. Musicians may get calluses on their fingers due to friction from guitar strings etc.

General Signs and Symptoms: There are 2 main types of corn. Hard corns are the most common. They show as small circles of hard skin with a clear centre, usually on bony parts of the toes. Soft corns are whitish and rubbery in texture and are usually found in areas between the toes. They can be extremely painful and are subject to infection due to their moist location. Calluses are yellowy, rough, usually painless areas of hard skin, occurring on areas of the feet and hands subjected to excess friction.

Conventional Medical Treatment: Removing the source of pressure or friction is a priority. Corn pads can be used to keep the pressure off a hard corn and a variety of toe separators and special plasters is available. A Doctor or Chiropodist may be able to cut off some of the hard callused skin or reduce the size of the corn by paring it down. Calluses can be gradually removed by soaking the feet in warm water and then gently rubbing them with a pumice stone.

Prognosis: Once the callus or corn has been removed it should not return providing that the source of the pressure or friction is also eliminated. Corns and calluses may become infected and ulcerated, particularly in those with diabetes. If this occurs, medical help should be sought.

Holistic Advice: Wear shoes that fit. Wash the feet regularly and dry them properly. Moisturising the feet with special foot cream may help. Change socks or tights every day.

Cough

Definition: A reflex response to an infection or irritation of the respiratory tract.

Possible Causes: Acute coughs are commonly caused by a viral infection of the respiratory tract, such as the common cold, flu, laryngitis or bronchitis. Allergic conditions (e.g. hay fever) may also cause a cough. The respiratory tract can also be irritated by mucus and inhaled irritants such as dust and smoke which cause the reflex action. Coughs can also be caused when small objects, typically pieces of food, are accidentally inhaled. Chronic coughs can be caused by smoking, underlying conditions (e.g. asthma, rhinitis and gastro-oesophageal reflux) and can be a side effect of some medicines (e.g. ACE inhibitors). Occasionally a cough can be a symptom of a more serious condition (e.g. lung cancer and heart failure).

General Signs and Symptoms: There are 2 main types of cough. A dry cough feels like a constant tickle in the throat and no phlegm is produced. A chesty or productive cough (usually as a result of infection) feels deeper and phlegm may be produced. The chest and ribs may become sore with the exertion of coughing and, because sleep may be affected (coughs tend to be worse when lying flat), the sufferer may feel tired and achy.

Conventional Medical Treatment: Cough medicines may help to relieve the symptoms. For dry coughs, cough suppressants may be used. For chesty coughs, expectorants may help bring up the phlegm so that coughing becomes easier. Antibiotics serve no purpose for viral infections, but may be prescribed if there is a secondary bacterial infection. If the condition persists, investigations such as X-rays or lung function tests may be required to ensure there is no serious underlying condition.

Prognosis: Most coughs only last a few days to a couple of weeks. If the cough produces bloody mucus or causes chest pain or shortness of breath, medical advice should be sought.

Holistic Advice: Lemon and honey drinks are useful to soothe the throat. Steam inhalation may help to loosen the mucus. Anything that can boost the immune system will be of benefit because the cough (if viral) will remain until the body defeats it.

Cramp

Definition: Sudden painful contraction of a muscle.

Possible Causes: Most cramps have no underlying cause, but they can be brought on by vigorous exercise, which causes an accumulation of lactic acid in the muscle. Excessive sweating can also lead to a loss of sodium which often causes cramp. Cramp may also be associated with poor circulation, or triggered by swimming in cold water, over-tiredness and tension. Occasionally, cramp may be an indication of an underlying disease such as motor neuron problems, metabolic problems such as liver, kidney or thyroid conditions, and dehydration. Certain medications may also induce leg cramps, e.g. diuretics, statins (used to lower blood-cholesterol levels) and some asthma drugs.

General Signs and Symptoms: Painful and sudden contraction of muscle, commonly in the legs. The calf is most often affected but the thigh and feet can get cramp too. Cramp can cause a lack of mobility and normally lasts only for a few seconds. After an episode of cramp, the muscle will often feel hard and painful and remain sore for several hours.

Conventional Medical Treatment: Because there is usually no underlying cause, treatment is very limited. Due to the speed and duration of the attacks, painkillers are unlikely to be of benefit. In some cases, quinine has shown to have benefits but more research is necessary, particularly regarding any side effects. Self-help is likely to be the best route. Stretching the muscles and massaging the affected muscle can bring relief.

Prognosis: Although unpleasant and sometimes very painful, cramp is not likely to cause any lasting damage. Exercises to stretch the muscles can help to prevent cramp as well as ease it out when it strikes.

Holistic Advice: For night cramp, keeping the feet warm can help, so use bed socks or place the feet on a feather pillow (which holds body heat and does not go cold like a hot water bottle). Supporting the toes while asleep may also help. A regular massage can be of benefit because it may stimulate the circulation and lymphatic system, helping to release tension and waste products from the muscles.

Crohn's Disease

Definition: A chronic inflammatory disease that can affect any part of the digestive tract.

Possible Causes: The exact cause is unknown. There may be a genetic factor, because there is more chance of developing Crohn's disease if close relatives have it. It may be caused by a malfunction in the immune system, causing the body to attack "friendly bacteria" in the intestines, and various environmental factors are also thought to play a part. Smokers are twice as likely to develop this disease than non-smokers, and their symptoms are often more severe.

General Signs and Symptoms: Areas of the digestive tract become inflamed. Any part of the digestive tract can be affected but it is most commonly found in the ileum and the colon. Inflammation often occurs in more than one part of the tract, with unaffected or mildly affected areas between. The inflammation can cause diarrhoea, abdominal pain, fever, weight loss and a general feeling of ill health. If the colon is affected the stools may contain blood and there may be some rectal bleeding. Episodes may be severe, lasting weeks or even months, before settling down to show only mild (or no) symptoms. Usually begins in early adulthood and can cause serious ill health throughout life.

Conventional Medical Treatment: Mild attacks can be treated with antidiarrhoeal drugs. For an acute attack steroids are commonly prescribed. Severe cases may need hospitalisation. Aminosalicylate drugs (to reduce persistent inflammation of the intestines) and immunosuppressant drugs may be prescribed to help reduce the frequency of the attacks. Dietary supplements may be required to counter any malabsorption. Most sufferers will need surgery at some stage to remove the diseased area.

Prognosis: Symptoms tend to recur despite treatment and the condition is lifelong. Complications such as intestinal obstruction, ulcers, fistulae (passageways that develop and run from the bowel), and malabsorption problems may occur. There is also a significantly increased risk of developing colorectal cancer.

Holistic Advice: Keep a food diary to see if any foods worsen the condition.

Cushing's Syndrome

Definition: Hormonal disorder associated with high levels of steroid hormones.

Possible Causes: Constantly high levels of steroid hormones in the blood. This could be due to long term treatment with steroid medication for another illness (e.g. asthma or arthritis), or a disorder that causes the overproduction of cortisol (e.g. pituitary or adrenal tumours).

General Signs and Symptoms: Sudden weight gain, bloating around the chest and stomach, red and rounded face, excessive growth of facial or body hair (especially in women), irregular menstruation or amenorrhoea, reddish-purple stretch marks on the abdomen, thighs, buttocks, breasts, arms and legs, oedema, heavy sweating, muscle wasting and weakness, tendency to bruise easily, wounds slow to heal, acne, loss of libido, depression and mood swings. Some may experience headaches, high blood pressure, high blood glucose level, an increased thirst and an increased need to urinate.

Conventional Medical Treatment: If it is caused by taking steroid medication for another illness, it may be possible to reduce the dose and seek alternative treatments. If the body is producing too much cortisol, cortisol-inhibiting drugs may be used. If the symptoms are caused by a tumour, the tumour may be removed by surgery, radiotherapy or chemotherapy, all of which have possible serious complications.

Prognosis: May be cured but recovery is slow. Untreated it can lead to complications such as high blood pressure, thinning of the bones, diabetes mellitus and chronic heart failure.

Holistic Advice: Never alter the dose of any prescribed drug without first consulting a doctor.

Cystitis

Definition: Inflammation of the bladder. Because the bladder is a part of the urinary tract, cystitis is classed as a urinary tract infection (UTI).

Possible Causes: Usually it is a result of a bacterial infection which causes inflammation of the bladder lining. Bacterial infection can be caused by not emptying the bladder fully (so harbouring bacteria), and by bacteria entering the urethra from the anal or vaginal areas and then travelling up to the bladder. Cystitis can also be caused by the irritation or damage to the area around the urethra. This can be caused by factors such as frequent or vigorous sex, wearing tight clothing and chemical irritants. It can also be symptomatic of some underlying conditions such as other bladders problems, kidney conditions and, in males, prostatitis. People with diabetes mellitus are more likely to suffer from urinary tract infections because the presence of glucose in the urine may encourage bacterial growth.

General Signs and Symptoms: The most common symptoms are an urgent and frequent need to urinate, and pain or stinging when passing urine. Other symptoms include dark, cloudy or strong smelling urine, a feeling of incomplete emptying of the bladder, blood in the urine, and lower abdominal pain. The sufferer may feel generally unwell, weak and feverish. Cystitis is more common in women than men and more frequent if the woman is pregnant, sexual active or post-menopausal.

Conventional Medical Treatment: Mild cystitis can often be cleared up by drinking plenty of water and taking painkillers such as paracetamol and ibuprofen. More serious infections may need antibiotics.

Prognosis: Most cases clear up on their own, but some do not respond to antibiotics and the sufferer may experience many recurring episodes. It is also possible for the infection to move to the kidneys. In a few severe cases, there can be a complete or partial loss of bladder control as a result of the irritation of the muscle in the bladder wall.

Holistic Advice: Avoid synthetic underwear, tights and close fitting trousers. Drink plenty of water and cranberry juice. Do not use any perfumed products around the genitals. Empty the bladder frequently and completely, after going to the toilet wipe from front to back, wash before and after sex, and urinate after sex. Avoid coffee, food containing vinegar, citrus fruits and spicy foods as these may trigger the condition.

Dandruff

Definition: Common condition that affects the scalp causing flakes of skin to appear.

Possible Causes: It is associated with the accelerated renewal of skin cells, which causes more dead skin to be shed. Sensitivity to yeasts that are produced naturally by the body can cause dandruff, and not brushing hair regularly results in the dead skin cells not being physically removed. Excessive dandruff is known as seborrhoeic dermatitis, which causes the skin to become inflamed and flaky, and results in larger, greasier flakes.

General Signs and Symptoms: White flakes of skin on the scalp and in the hair. Head may feel sore, greasy or itchy. Affects men more than women, often after puberty.

Conventional Medical Treatment: Dandruff shampoos and scalp preparations can be used to control the condition. Antifungal shampoos inhibit the growth of the fungi and yeasts. In severe cases the GP may prescribe steroid scalp applications to reduce the inflammation.

Prognosis: Responds well to treatment but can reoccur at any time.

Holistic Advice: Although not caused by poor hygiene, it can affect self-esteem. Ensure hair is rinsed properly after washing and brush hair regularly. Avoid using chemicals on the scalp. Try to keep well hydrated to avoid the skin from drying.

Deep Vein Thrombosis

Definition: Formation of a blood clot within a deep lying vein, usually in the leg. Often abbreviated to DVT. Also called venous thrombosis.

Possible Causes: Usually caused by a combination of slow blood flow through a vein, an increased tendency of the blood to clot, and a damaged vein wall. Risk factors include long periods of immobility (e.g. during a long air flight or if confined to bed), pregnancy, accidental injury to a blood vessel, surgery, family history of thrombosis, being overweight, smoking, dehydration and taking the combined oral contraceptive pill.

General Signs and Symptoms: Pain or tenderness in the leg, swelling of the lower leg or thigh, enlarged veins below the skin, heavy ache in the affected limb and redness and heat in the affected area.

Conventional Medical Treatment: Anticoagulants, such as heparin and warfarin, may be used to help prevent the clot getting bigger and to reduce the risk of further clots developing. Compression stockings can help prevent the calf from swelling and reduce the pain. Only rarely is surgery used to remove a clot. Raising the leg above the hip helps to relieve the pressure on the vein.

Prognosis: DVT is not usually dangerous in itself, but there is a risk that a fragment of the clot could break off and lodge in a pulmonary artery, causing a pulmonary embolism. A history of DVT may lead to post-thrombotic syndrome, causing long term symptoms such as calf pain, swelling, a rash in the affected area and (in severe cases) ulcers.

Holistic Advice: Try to avoid long periods of inactivity. Stretch and move regularly. Take regular exercise, lose any excess weight, don't smoke and eat a healthy diet. Drink plenty of water.

Depression

Definition: Feelings of sadness, often accompanied by loss of interest in life and reduced energy. It is one of the most common mental health disorders. Specific types of depression exist, including seasonal affective disorder, postnatal depression, and bipolar depression (manic depression), in which there are periods of depression and periods of excessively high mood (mania).

Possible Causes: There is no single cause. It can be triggered by a stressful event (or more commonly a combination of stressful events) such as bereavement, divorce, illness, and job and money worries. Risk factors include certain conditions such as coronary heart disease, cancer, and head injuries, low self esteem, family history of depression, traumatic event in childhood, giving birth, social isolation, drinking alcohol and taking drugs. Women are more likely than men to become depressed but, given that the suicide rate in men is higher, this could be because men are less likely to seek help for their depression.

General Signs and Symptoms: Feeling of sadness or misery that lasts most of the day. Common symptoms include loss of interest and motivation, low energy, tearfulness, poor concentration, low self-esteem, feeling worried or anxious, feelings of guilt, difficulty in making decisions, insomnia, unexplained aches and pains, loss of hope, changes in appetite and weight, and decreased sex drive. There may be thoughts about self-harm or suicide. Depression can interfere with working, social and family lives.

Conventional Medical Treatment: Mild depression can often spontaneously lift. Antidepressants may be prescribed and psychosocial treatments (such as counselling and cognitive behavioural therapy) used. For severe depression, electroconvulsive therapy or lithium may be recommended. Depression may recur if antidepressant drugs are withdrawn too soon.

Prognosis: With the right treatment and support, most make a full recovery.

Holistic Advice: Take regular exercise and maintain a balanced, healthy diet. Try to talk about feelings with others. Relaxation techniques and breathing exercises may help, as may engaging in a distracting hobby. Support groups can offer advice and information, as well as providing a forum to openly discuss feelings with those who have had similar experiences. There are many self-help books, CDs and DVDs to help with depression. Always remember that depression is a serious illness, not a weakness.

Diabetes Insipidus

Definition: Disorder caused by the body's inability to control its water balance. Not related to diabetes mellitus, although both conditions cause thirst and the excessive passing of urine.

Possible Causes: The amount of water in the body is regulated by antidiuretic hormone (ADH). In this condition either too little is produced (cranial diabetes insipidus) or the body fails to respond to its effect (nephrogenic diabetes insipidus). This results in too much urine being passed which, in turn, causes the extreme thirst. The most common cause of cranial diabetes insipidus is damage to the hypothalamus caused by a brain tumour, brain surgery or a head injury. It may also be caused by the immune system attacking brain tissue. Other causes include cancers that spread to the brain, brain infections that cause damage and conditions that suddenly reduce the blood supply to the brain (e.g. stroke). Nephrogenic diabetes insipidus may be congenital or acquired. The most common cause of acquired nephrogenic diabetes insipidus is taking certain medications (e.g. lithium (used for bipolar disorder)). Other causes include having too much calcium in the blood or too little potassium, and kidney damage caused by infection or obstruction.

General Signs and Symptoms: There is a persistent thirst and the frequent need to pass a large quantity of pale, dilute urine. These symptoms can affect sleeping patterns, causing tiredness and irritability. Sufferers may feel generally unwell.

Conventional Medical Treatment: Treatment aims to reduce the quantity of urine passed. Cranial diabetes insipidus may be treated with a drug called desmopressin that mimics antidiuretic hormone. Thiazide diuretics may be used to increase the concentration of the urine which, in these cases, decreases the output. Non-steroidal anti-inflammatory drugs may also help. Nephrogenic diabetes insipidus may be treated by a change of medication. A change of diet is also commonly required. Thiazide diuretics and non-steroidal anti-inflammatory drugs may be prescribed in severe cases. It is important to drink sufficiently so as not to become dehydrated.

Prognosis: Outlook depends on the cause.

Holistic Advice: Sufferers should carry identification to alert others of the condition in case of emergency.

Diabetes Mellitus

Definition: Chronic condition caused by too much glucose in the blood. There are 2 types of diabetes mellitus - type 1 and type 2 (see below).

Possible Causes: The amount of sugar in the blood is controlled by insulin. Insulin helps to move glucose from the blood into the cells to be broken down to release energy. Type 1 diabetes occurs when no insulin is produced. Type 1 usually occurs suddenly in childhood and is often referred to as juvenile diabetes or early-onset diabetes. It is thought to be an autoimmune condition in which the cells of the pancreas are attacked. This may be triggered by a viral infection, and there may be a familial link. In type 2 diabetes, either too little insulin is secreted or the body's cells become resistant to it, and so the glucose in the blood in not fully utilized. About 95% of all diabetics have this type. It develops slowly but the exact cause is not known. The risk of type 2 diabetes increases with age and is linked to obesity. Ethnic origin may be a factor (African-Caribbean or south Asian origins are more at risk) and it appears to be familial.

General Signs and Symptoms: Deposits of sugar in the urine, extreme thirst and a dry mouth, increased urination, constipation, lack of energy, dehydrated skin, recurring thrush, blurred vision, cramps, muscle weakness, loss of weight, skin infections and poor circulation, which can result in wounds being slow to heal. If the blood sugar becomes very low, a "hypo" attack may occur causing the sufferer to feel shaky, sweaty, weak, sick and confused.

Conventional Medical Treatment: The aim of treatment is to keep blood glucose levels as normal as possible. Type 1 diabetes is treated with insulin injections and so is often referred to as insulin dependent diabetes. Type 2 can usually be controlled at first by adapting the diet and making lifestyle changes. If the blood glucose level creeps up, oral medicines can be given to reduce it but insulin injections may be required ultimately. A hypo attack is treated by giving sugar orally or a glucagon injection to raise the blood glucose level.

Prognosis: There is no cure and it is a lifelong condition. Complications can cause eye, kidney, cardiovascular and nervous system problems. Blood glucose levels, blood pressure and cholesterol levels should be regularly monitored.

Holistic Advice: Exercise regularly and lose excess weight. Don't smoke. Only drink alcohol in moderation. A usual healthy diet that is high in fibre, fruit and vegetable and low in fat, salt and sugar is advised. Diabetes dietitians offer specific advice. Take care of the feet and eyes, and information cards should be carried or a bracelet worn if prone to unstable blood sugar levels.

Diarrhoea

Definition: The passing of frequent, loose watery stools.

Possible Causes: Diarrhoea is not a disease in itself but may be a symptom of an underlying condition. Short (acute) bouts, especially if accompanied by vomiting, are often caused by gastroenteritis. Gastroenteritis is commonly caused by a viral infection (e.g. norovirus) or bacterial infection (e.g. E.coli and salmonella). Those with reduced immunity are more susceptible to infectious gastroenteritis. Other causes of acute diarrhoea include emotional upset, taking antibiotics, and drinking too much alcohol or coffee. Chronic diarrhoea, lasting more than 2 weeks, can also be due to a viral or bacterial infection, but can also be caused by the use of laxatives, poor diet, or can be symptomatic of an underlying intestinal disorder, e.g. ulcerative colitis, irritable bowel syndrome, Crohn's disease and lactose intolerance.

General Signs and Symptoms: Diarrhoea may be accompanied by abdominal pain, bloating, loss of appetite and vomiting. Can lead to dehydration, causing headache, weakness and lethargy.

Conventional Medical Treatment: Usually clears up within a couple of days. Drink plenty of water. Associated symptoms tend to clear when rehydrated. Rehydration drinks can help rebalance the salt and sugar levels. Antidiarrhoeal drugs can help reduce the bowel movement but are not always advised. Painkillers can help any fever or headache. If caused by an underlying intestinal disorder, the disorder will be addressed.

Prognosis: Usually temporary, but if prolonged the underlying cause must be established. Dehydration can be dangerous, particularly in babies, children and the elderly.

Holistic Advice: The risk of developing infectious gastroenteritis (and therefore diarrhoea) can be reduced by washing the hands regularly, particularly after going to the toilet and before eating.

Diverticular Disease

Definition: The presence of small pouches known as diverticula in the wall of the colon that cause the symptoms associated with this disease.

Possible Causes: Pea-sized pouches form when parts of the intestine (usually the lower colon) bulge outwards. The bulging is often associated with persistent constipation. It is estimated that by the age of 50, 50% of people will have diverticula. When the presence of these pouches causes symptoms, it is called diverticular disease. When the pouches become infected and inflamed (possibly by a hard piece of faeces getting trapped in the pouch, allowing bacteria to develop) the condition is called diverticulitis. Risk factors may include low-fibre diet, smoking, obesity, having a history of constipation, physical inactivity, and the use of non-steroidal anti-inflammatory drugs (e.g. ibuprofen).

General Signs and Symptoms: Diverticular disease can cause episodes of abdominal pain (especially in the lower left abdomen) and bloating that is relieved by defaecation or the passing of wind. There may be intermittent bouts of constipation and diarrhoea, and occasional bright red bleeding from the rectum. Diverticulitis can cause a more persistent, severe lower abdominal pain, tenderness in the abdomen, fever, nausea, vomiting, painful or frequent urination, and rectal bleeding.

Conventional Medical Treatment: Often a high-fibre diet with plenty of fluids is the only treatment required for diverticular disease. Paracetamol tends to be recommended for the abdominal pain. Diverticulitis may require antibiotics to treat any bacterial infection. Surgery may be required to remove the diseased part of the colon if severe bouts of diverticulitis occur frequently.

Prognosis: Diverticular disease can usually be controlled and does not have serious associated complications. However, with diverticulitis, the inflamed diverticula can burst, allowing faeces and blood to spill into the abdominal cavity. This can lead to peritonitis (the inflammation of the lining of the abdomen), which can be fatal if not treated quickly. There is also the risk of abscesses, fistulae (passageways that develop and run from the bowel) and intestinal obstruction.

Holistic Advice: Drink plenty of fluids and eat a high-fibre diet. Any changes in bowel movement or rectal bleeding should be reported to a Doctor as it can indicate a serious underlying disease.

Dysmenorrhoea

Definition: Pain associated with menstruation.

Possible Causes: In most cases the pain is a normal part of the menstrual cycle, caused by muscular contractions of the uterine wall. This is called primary dysmenorrhoea and there may be a familial link. In some cases, dysmenorrhoea is caused by an underlying medical condition such as endometriosis, fibroids, pelvic inflammatory disease, adenomyosis (when the uterine lining grows into the muscular layer of the uterus) and having an intrauterine contraceptive device fitted. This is called secondary dysmenorrhoea.

General Signs and Symptoms: Pain and/or painful cramping in the lower abdomen. The pain may radiate to the lower back and legs. Other symptoms may include headache, nausea, tiredness, dizziness and diarrhoea. The symptoms usually begin just before or at the start of menstruation, with the pain being worst when the bleeding is heaviest.

Conventional Medical Treatment: Primary dysmenorrhoea may be treated with over-the-counter non-steroidal anti-inflammatory drugs (e.g. ibuprofen and aspirin) or other pain killers such as paracetamol. The use of the combined contraceptive pill may also help to reduce symptoms. In cases of secondary dysmenorrhoea, the underlying condition will be treated. Once under control, the dysmenorrhoea usually disappears.

Prognosis: Can usually be successfully treated.

Holistic Advice: Taking hot baths or applying a source of heat to the abdomen (e.g. hot water bottle) may provide relief. Gentle exercise may help to reduce the pain. Light circular massage around the abdomen may be helpful. Relaxation techniques may also be of benefit.

Ear Problems

General Information: Disorders of the ear are very common and in severe cases may interfere with communication, causing significant disability. As well as being the organs of hearing, the inner ear also contains structures that help to maintain balance and so disorders of the ear can lead to symptoms such as dizziness. Below is a brief summary of 5 common ear conditions.

Deafness: Partial or total loss of hearing in one or both ears. May be congenital, or caused by disease, injury or age. Deafness that results from the failure of the outer ear to transmit sound to the inner ear is often temporary, e.g. when the middle ear fills with fluid following infection or wax, or sudden changes in air pressure. Damage to the part of the inner ear that detects sound or to the nerve tends to cause permanent deafness, e.g. noise-induced hearing loss or Ménière's disease (a disorder of the inner ear causing sudden episodes of severe dizziness, nausea and hearing loss). Hearing aids are commonly used to help correct permanent deafness.

Earache: Pain originating in the ear. It can be caused by a wide range of ear disorders, infections and blockages, but can also be caused by the build up of mucus after a cold or toothache.

Glue Ear: Childhood condition in which fluid builds up in the middle ear. It causes temporary, partial deafness but usually gets better without medical intervention.

Tinnitus: Sounds, often ringing, buzzing or whistling, that originate from one or both ears. The sounds may vary in volume, and episodes can be brief but in some it is permanent. Cause is often unknown but can be associated with ear disorders such as Ménière's disease and noise-induced hearing loss. It may also be a symptom of an underlying medical condition, e.g. anaemia and hyperthyroidism. Masking devices can be used that produce sounds to distract from the tinnitus. It can be very distressing, leading to depression and anxiety.

Vertigo: A false sensation of movement, often combined with nausea and vomiting. It may be impossible to walk or even stand. Vertigo often develops suddenly, lasting a few seconds to several days. It is caused by a disturbance in the inner ear resulting from many factors including arthritis in the neck (that affects blood flow to parts of the brain associated with balance), inner ear infections, Ménière's disease, excess alcohol, heatstroke and food poisoning. Lying still will help in the short term. The underlying cause must be identified for persistent episodes.

Emphysema

Definition: Progressive damage to the lungs, resulting in wheezing and shortness of breath. Sufferers also usually have chronic bronchitis and the resulting condition is called chronic obstructive pulmonary disease (COPD).

Possible Causes: In emphysema the alveoli in the lungs become enlarged and damaged, making them less efficient in transferring oxygen to the blood stream. In chronic bronchitis the bronchi become inflamed, congested and narrowed, obstructing the flow of air. Smoking is the most common cause. Air pollution, passive smoking, and occupational exposure to fumes, dust and other lung irritants, can be contributory factors. Smokers with a sibling with COPD are at a higher risk of developing the disease, and there is a rare genetic condition that causes a deficiency of a protein that protects the lungs, so increasing the risk of COPD.

General Signs and Symptoms: Difficulty breathing, wheezing and shortness of breath. The symptoms build up gradually, getting worse over time. There tends to be a persistent productive cough, an increase in sputum production and frequent chest infections. Cold weather and infections such as flu worsen the condition. Some sufferers of emphysema may develop a barrel-shaped chest as the lungs distend. It is more common in men although the incidence in women is rising.

Conventional Medical Treatment: Damage to the lungs caused by COPD is irreversible. Preventing further exposure by making lifestyle changes as soon as possible is the only way to limit further damage. Treatment can only help ease the symptoms. Bronchodilator drugs can help make breathing easier, mucolytic drugs can help thin the mucus to make it easier to cough up. Antibiotics may be used to help treat chest infections and steroids may be prescribed for a bad flare-up. In severe cases nebulisers (to administer medicine in vapour form through a face mask) and oxygen therapy may be required. If fluid builds up in the tissues, diuretics may be prescribed.

Prognosis: It can result in respiratory failure, reduced kidney function and heart failure. Fewer than 1 in 20 people with COPD live longer than 10 years after diagnosis.

Holistic Advice: Stop smoking. Take gentle exercise. Vaccinations against flu and pneumonia may be recommended.

Endometriosis

Definition: The presence of endometrium cells (the cells that line the interior wall of the uterus) in other parts of the body, such as the fallopian tubes, ovaries, bladder, bowel, vagina and rectum.

Possible Causes: The endometriosis cells outside of the womb go through a menstrual pattern in the same way as the endometrium. However, when these cells break down causing a bleed, the blood is trapped in the body. This can lead to pain, swelling and tissue damage. The cause is not known for certain, but it may be caused by fragments of the endometrium which, when shed during menstruation, do not leave the body as normal, but instead travel along the fallopian tubes, possibly enter the pelvic cavity and attach to organs. It may also be the case that endometriosis cells travel to other parts of the body by accessing the blood or lymphatic systems. It may also be caused by a combination of genetic, immune system, hormonal and environmental factors.

General Signs and Symptoms: Pain in the lower abdomen, pelvis or lower back, particularly before and during menstrual periods. Menorrhagia (excessive menstrual flow), dysmenorrhoea (painful menstruation) and irregular menstruation are common. Sufferers may have a lack of energy, depression, fertility problems and experience pain during sexual intercourse. The pain varies according to where the cells are located.

Conventional Medical Treatment: In mild cases the condition may get better by itself. The pain can be reduced with non-steroidal anti-inflammatories and pain killers. Hormone treatments can be given for several months to limit or stop the production of oestrogen and so prevent menstruation. This may help reduce the endometriosis. Surgery can be used to remove or destroy areas of endometriosis tissue, depending on where the tissue is located. In severe cases, a hysterectomy and the removal of the ovaries plus any areas of endometriosis may be suggested.

Prognosis: It is a chronic condition with no cure but symptoms can usually be managed successfully. Infertility is the greatest problem and, although some treatments may increase fertility, getting pregnant can often be problematic. Adhesions on the ovaries may also lead to ovarian cysts. Endometriosis may recur until the menstrual cycle ends at the menopause, but is unlikely to recur if the ovaries are removed.

Holistic Advice: Relaxation exercises can be useful to help to cope with the pain.

Epilepsy

Definition: A disorder of brain function causing recurrent seizures.

Possible Causes: Seizures are symptomatic of abnormal electrical activity in the brain. There are 3 main types. 1. Symptomatic - when there is a known cause (e.g. brain injury, drug or alcohol abuse, meningitis, stroke and brain tumour). 2. Idiopathic – when there is no known cause. 3. Cryptogenic – when there is no known cause but there is evidence (such as learning disorders) to suggest that it may be due to brain damage. Triggers may include stress, lack of sleep, fever, low blood-sugar level, and flashing lights.

General Signs and Symptoms: Seizures vary from a few seconds in a trance-like state, to convulsions and total loss of consciousness. Seizures are categorized according to how much of the brain is affected. In a partial seizure, only a part of the brain is affected but a generalised seizure affects all (or most) of the brain. Partial seizures may be simple or complex. In a simple partial seizure, consciousness is maintained but the head and eyes may turn to one side, the muscles in the arms, legs and face may stiffen, and one side of the body may twitch. There may be tingling sensations, muscle weakness and strange sensory sensations. In a complex partial seizure, the person may enter an uncommunicative state. They may smack the lips, grimace and fidget, and have no memory of the seizure. A generalised seizure may render the person unconscious and often leads to a fall. There are several types including absences (loss of awareness, most common in children), myoclonic jerks (muscle twitches), clonic seizure (longer lasting twitching), atonic seizure (causing all the muscles to relax), tonic seizure (causing all the muscles to stiffen) and tonic-clonic seizure. Tonic-clonic seizure is the most common form of epilepsy. It is typified by body stiffness, twitchy limbs, loss of consciousness and urinary incontinence. Epileptics may be able to feel the onset of an episode

Conventional Medical Treatment: Most cases can be successfully treated with anti-epileptic drugs. Failing that, vagus nerve stimulation may be considered. A device is implanted that stimulates the vagus nerve in the neck. This has been shown to reduce the frequency and severity of the attacks. Brain surgery is only used if the part of the brain affected is small and its removal would not cause a significant loss of brain function.

Prognosis: There in no cure but treatments can usually control the condition.

Holistic Advice: Because stress may trigger an attack, exercise and relaxation exercises such as yoga and meditation may help. Avoid all triggers.

Eye Problems

General Information: Many eye disorders do not affect sight but a few serious conditions may damage the structures of the eye and lead to loss of vision. Eye disorders are common and early diagnosis tends to lead to successful treatment.

Cataract: Clouding of the lens of the eye, causing blurred or distorted vision. The cataracts are caused by structural changes to protein fibres in the lens, resulting in the cloudy appearance. They can be congenital but are most common after the age of 75. They usually develop in both eyes but one can be more severely affected. Risk factors for cataracts in the young are eye injury, prolonged exposure to sunlight, diabetes mellitus, or long term use of corticosteroids. The cataract can be surgically removed and an artificial lens put into the eye.

Corneal Ulcer: A deep erosion of the cornea. Corneal ulcers can be very painful and, if left untreated, can cause scarring and lead to permanently impaired vision, blindness or even loss of the eye. They can be caused by injury and/or infection. Symptoms include intense pain in the eye, redness and discharge from the eye, and an increased sensitivity to light. People who wear contact lenses are at increased risk. Antibiotics or antiviral drugs may be prescribed to treat the infection, which usually clears up with 1-2 weeks.

Glaucoma: Abnormally high pressure of fluid inside the eye. This is caused by a blockage of the fluid as it tries naturally to flow out of the eye. The rise in pressure may cause damage to the nerve fibres in the retina (the light-sensitive part of the eye) and the optic nerve causing permanent damage. It mainly affects those over 60 and is familial. Glaucoma can be acute (developing suddenly, causing severe pain and rapid loss of vision) or chronic (developing painlessly over several years). It is diagnosed by measuring the eye pressure. Eye drops can be used to reduce the pressure. In some cases surgery may be needed to help the fluid drain. Successful treatment normally minimizes further vision loss but if left untreated it can cause blindness.

Female Infertility

Definition: Inability of a woman to conceive with a partner of normal fertility.

Possible Causes: There are 3 main stages to conception – ovulation, egg transport and fertilization, and implantation. Infertility can be caused by problems with any of these, but is most commonly caused by problems with ovulation. Conditions such as polycystic ovary syndrome, premature menopause, thyroid disorders, and some chronic conditions (such as cancer) may affect ovulation. Damage to the fallopian tubes and uterus affect successful egg transport, fertilization and implantation. Damage can be caused by a variety factors, including pelvic or cervical surgery, fibroids, endometriosis, and pelvic inflammatory disease. Risk factors include stress, excessive exercise, low body weight, obesity, some medications, age, sexually transmitted infections, smoking, and exposure to some chemicals.

General Signs and Symptoms: Inability to conceive despite having regular unprotected sex.

Conventional Medical Treatment: Medication can be given to encourage ovulation, surgical procedures may be used to help correct any anatomical problem, and assisted conception techniques, such as intrauterine insemination and in-vitro fertilization, can help sperm to fertilize the egg. When fertility can not be helped by any of the above treatments, it may be possible to receive donated eggs.

Prognosis: Treatments significantly increase the chance of pregnancy, but the success rates vary depending on the cause of infertility and the treatment given.

Holistic Advice: Infertility can put much stress on the woman and the relationship, which can then have the knock-on effect of further reducing the chances of conception. Try to reduce stress, use relaxation techniques, take regular, gentle exercise, eat a balanced diet, maintain a healthy weight, stop smoking, and avoid alcohol and illegal drugs. Folic acid supplements may be advised.

Fibroids

Definition: Non-cancerous tumours that grow slowly within the muscular wall of the uterus or around the uterus.

Possible Causes: Fibroids are abnormal growths of muscular and fibrous tissue, occurring singly or in groups. Fibroids can vary in size from the size of a pea to the size of a melon. They are found in about 1 in 4 women of childbearing age and are more common in Afro-Caribbeans. The cause of fibroids is unknown, but they are thought to be linked to the response of the uterus to oestrogen. This link is likely to be the reason why fibroids tend to grow at times of high oestrogen level and shrink after the menopause when the oestrogen level falls. The likelihood of fibroids increases with obesity.

General Signs and Symptoms: Many with small fibroids do not display any symptoms. The symptoms of larger fibroids may vary according to their size and location. Fibroids may cause prolonged and heavy menstrual bleeding, abdominal pain, abdominal swelling, back pain, the need to pass urine frequently, constipation, and pain or discomfort during sex.

Conventional Medical Treatment: Small fibroids may not need treatment but should be checked regularly to monitor any growth. Medication can be given to reduce oestrogen levels and to treat heavy menstrual flow. A hysterectomy may be necessary in cases of large fibroids and heavy bleeding. Fibroids may also be removed by a procedure called myomectomy, the lining of the uterus can be removed by endometrial ablation, and the blood vessels that feed the fibroids can be blocked in a procedure called uterine artery embolisation.

Prognosis: Generally fibroids shrink and disappear on their own, but sometimes they can cause pain and heavy bleeding and therefore require treatment. They can affect fertility.

Holistic Advice: Eat a balanced low-oestrogen diet and exercise regularly. Acupuncture and the Bowen Technique may be of benefit.

Fibromyalgia

Definition: A chronic (long term) condition that causes pain all over the body. Also called fibromyalgia syndrome.

Possible Causes: Exact cause is unknown but it has been shown that sufferers of fibromyalgia have a problem with the way in which pain messages are carried, have lower than normal levels of the hormones serotonin, noradrenaline and dopamine, and experience sleep problems. Triggers may also include physical or psychological trauma, viral infections, depression, metabolic disturbances such as an under-active thyroid, and inflammatory diseases such as rheumatoid arthritis. There may also be a genetic predisposition to this condition.

General Signs and Symptoms: Although the literal definition of the condition indicates pain (-algia) just in fibrous tissues (fibro-) and muscles (my-), the usual continuous pain extends all over the body, coupled with extreme fatigue. The condition may cause hyper-sensitivity to pain, so that even the slightest touch is painful. Stiffness, muscle spasms, poor quality of sleep, cognitive problems, headaches, and irritable bowel syndrome can also be associated. Severity of the symptoms may be affected by factors such as changes in the weather, stress levels and physical activity. Understandably, this condition often leads to depression. Affects women more than men, usually between the ages of 30-60 years

Conventional Medical Treatment: Currently no cure. Antidepressants, painkillers, muscle relaxants, anticonvulsants, antipsychotics, and medication to promote sleep can help alleviate the symptoms. Counselling-based therapies and lifestyle changes to promote good sleeping habits and relaxation can help, as may a tailored exercise programme.

Prognosis: For most the condition is permanent, but the symptoms vary in severity.

Holistic Advice: Network groups for this condition may be of use. Acupuncture, physiotherapy and treatments to aid relaxation may be of benefit. Balance periods of activity with periods of rest, don't overdo it, and rest when need to.

Flatulence

Definition: Passing of gas from the digestive system out of the anus.

Possible Causes: Every time food, drink or saliva is swallowed a small amount of air is ingested too. Gas is also released during the digestive process. This gas builds up in the digestive system and is released either through the mouth by belching or through the anus by flatulence. Food stuffs containing unabsorbable carbohydrates create more gas than other food. This is because these carbohydrates are not absorbed by the small intestine during the digestive process but get passed down to the colon where they get broken down by bacteria. This process produces gas. Foods that are high in unabsorbable carbohydrates include beans, cabbage and cauliflower. Some medical conditions can cause flatulence, e.g. constipation, irritable bowel syndrome, coeliac disease and lactose intolerance.

General Signs and Symptoms: Flatulence is a normal biological process and is only usually considered to be troublesome if there are frequent bouts of excessive wind and if the wind is considered to have a particularly unpleasant odour.

Conventional Medical Treatment: A dietary change is usually sufficient. Charcoal tablets can be purchased over-the-counter. The charcoal absorbs gas from the digestive system and so reduces flatulence.

Prognosis: Not considered to be harmful but if excessive flatulence occurs with other symptoms such as abdominal pain, bloating, episodes of constipation or diarrhoea, incontinence or blood in the stools, medical advice should be sought as it may be indicative of an underlying medical condition.

Holistic Advice: Smoking and chewing gum increases the amount of air swallowed, so avoiding these may help. Take regular exercise to promote a healthy digestive system. Peppermint tea may help.

Folliculitis

Definition: Inflammation of one or more hair follicles.

Possible Causes: Bacterial infection is the most common cause, but this is often preceded by physical damage to the follicle (e.g. friction, insect bite, shaving, blocked follicle). Sometimes associated with anaemia.

General Signs and Symptoms: Itchy or painful redness. Small red pimples develop in the upper part of the follicles which may then crust over. It can develop in any hairy areas of the body but is more common on the scalp, legs, buttocks, groin and armpits. In severe cases the infection may move further down into the skin creating larger areas of inflammation, even causing boils and widespread cellulitis (the bacterial infection of the dermis and subcutaneous layers of the skin). When present on the beard area of the face, folliculitis is known as Barber's itch. Pseudofolliculitis barbae is a disorder that occurs if curly beard hairs are cut too short, causing the hairs to curve back into the skin causing damage and subsequent inflammation.

Conventional Medical Treatment: Antiseptic lotions, creams and soaps are often sufficient to treat mild cases. Antibiotic creams applied topically can help to fight the infection. Antibiotic tablets may be required for stubborn infections.

Prognosis: Responds well to treatment. In severe cases it can cause scarring and, if the follicle is damaged, permanent hair loss.

Holistic Advice: Try to avoid further damage and irritation to the susceptible areas. Take extra care to ensure the infection is not spread by thoroughly cleaning equipment (e.g. razors) that makes contact with the vulnerable areas.

Foot Disorders

General Information: Feet are a weight bearing part of the body. Disorders affecting the feet can affect mobility and posture, and so have a knock-on affect to other parts of the musculoskeletal system. Here is a summary of 5 common skeletal foot disorders:

Bone Spur: A bone spur is an excessive formation of bone on normal bone. It is usually caused by localised inflammation, which triggers bone cells to deposit in the area. Spurs may cause pain if they rub surrounding tissue, and are commonly found in the back of the heel or the sole of the heel.

Club Foot: Congenital deformity of the ankle and foot. The foot (or both feet) points down and inwards. In mild cases no treatment will be necessary, but otherwise a technique called the Ponseti Method may be used to manipulate the foot into a better position and it is then set in a cast until the next manipulation is required. Surgery may also be needed to release the Achilles tendon.

Flat Feet: No space or only a little space between the foot and the ground under the medial longitudinal arch when standing. Also referred to as fallen arches. This can cause the foot to roll over to the inner side. It can be congenital but can also be caused by arthritis, a ruptured tendon, and muscular and nervous disorders. It can cause foot pain and stiffness but can often be corrected by wearing specially fitted insoles. Surgery may be required.

Foot Drop: The inability to raise the front part of the foot due to muscle weakness or paralysis caused by an underlying problem. When walking, the sufferer either drags the toes or has to lift the knee higher than normal to avoid doing so. It can be temporary or permanent, depending on the cause.

Hammer Toe: Deformity of the toe in which the end is bent downwards, so looking claw-like. Can be congenital or appear over time, sometimes caused by ill-fitting shoes. Initially it may be helped by exercising the joint to try to maintain and restore movement, but once it stiffens surgery may be necessary if it causes a problem.

High Arch: The opposite of flat foot, but much less common. The medial longitudinal arch is higher than usual, often causing pain. It is usually caused by a skeletal or nervous disorder.

<u>Fractures</u>

Definition: A break or crack in a bone. A simple (or closed) fracture is a clean break that has not damaged any surrounding tissues. A compound (or open) fracture is when the surrounding tissue and skin is damaged.

Possible Causes: Fractures are commonly caused by a bone being subjected to abnormal force due to, for example, a fall or accident. The bones weaken with age and so in later life bones break more easily. Diseases such as osteoporosis cause bones to thin and therefore make them more prone to fractures. Bone strength can also be decreased by certain infections, tumours and cysts. Fractures caused by underlying disease are called pathological fractures. Repeated small stresses and strains can cause stress fractures, common in athletes.

General Signs and Symptoms: Pain, swelling, misshapen body part, inability to bear weight, a grinding sound or sensation, or bleeding (in the case of an open fracture). The pain and shock may cause the sufferer to look pale, clammy and feel dizzy or sick.

Conventional Medical Treatment: The bones need to be realigned and held in place for the healing process to be effective. The bone may be able to be manipulated into shape or surgery may be required to reset the bone. Bones are commonly held in place by plaster casts, but other means such as plates, rods, pins etc, can be used externally and internally as appropriate.

Prognosis: Most bones that have been successfully realigned and immobilized for up to about 8 weeks heal successfully. Physiotherapy may be required afterwards to help rebuild muscular strength.

Holistic Advice: Bone strength can be helped by ensuring a balanced diet that includes calcium. Good sources of calcium include milk, cheese, yoghurt and green leafy vegetables. Vitamin D, formed naturally by the skin when exposed to sunlight, helps the body to absorb calcium. Vitamin D is also found in eggs and oily fish. Weight-bearing exercise can help strengthen the bones. Give up smoking.

Frozen Shoulder

Definition: Pain and restriction of movement in the shoulder joint.

Possible Causes: The capsule of the shoulder joint thickens, swells and tightens, making movement difficult and painful. The cause is not always known, but it can be due to inflammation resulting from an injury, or long-term immobility. It is more common in women than men and most frequently affects those between the ages of 40-60. Risk factors include diabetes, heart disease, lung disease, hyperthyroidism, Parkinson's disease and stroke.

General Signs and Symptoms: Pain and stiffness in the shoulder joint. The condition usually starts with aching and stiffness and then it causes severe pain. The stiffness worsens and muscle tone can be lost due to the lack of movement. The pain may radiate to the elbow and be worse at night.

Conventional Medical Treatment: Painkillers or non-steroidal anti-inflammatory drugs may be prescribed to relieve the pain and reduce inflammation. Corticosteroid injections to the shoulder may be used and physiotherapy may be required. Surgery is rarely used but is an option should all other treatments be unsuccessful.

Prognosis: Recovery can be slow - even taking several years - but most regain full movement.

Holistic Advice: It is important to keep as much movement as possible in the shoulder. Acupuncture claims to be effective in some cases. Bowen may possibly bring relief for some too.

Gallstones

Definition: Small stones that form in the gall bladder.

Possible Causes: It is thought that gallstones develop due to an imbalance in the chemical composition of bile. Gallstones are commonly made up of cholesterol and so a diet high in cholesterol may be a cause. Risk factors include age, sex (women are more likely to develop stones), obesity, cirrhosis and family history.

General Signs and Symptoms: Gallstones are present in about 1 in 10 people but usually go unnoticed. This is called asymptomatic gallstones. However, sudden and intense pain in the abdomen, nausea, vomiting and sweating (a collection of symptoms called biliary colic) may be experienced if stones become trapped and block a duct. This is called uncomplicated gallstones and usually lasts 1-5 hours. Complicated gallstones is the most serious, and occurs when the gallstones cause inflammation of the gall bladder, bile ducts or pancreas. These inflammatory conditions are associated with a high temperature and symptoms that last more than 8 hours. Complicated gallstones can be very serious and medical advice should be sought without delay.

Conventional Medical Treatment: The most effective treatment is to remove the gall bladder, but in mild cases the symptoms may not recur frequently and so surgery may not be necessary. Reducing the amount of fat in the diet may help and painkillers can be used during an attack. Less effective treatments include removing the gallstones but not the gall bladder, using drugs to dissolve the gallstones (if they are made of cholesterol) and using ultrasonic shock waves to break up the stones.

Prognosis: Removal of the gall bladder usually cures the problem. If the gall bladder is not removed there is an ongoing risk of recurrent attacks or gallstones reforming.

Holistic Advice: Eat a low fat, high fibre diet, lose any excess weight and take regular exercise.

Ganglion

Definition: A fluid-filled cyst that develops around joints and tendons.

Possible Causes: Arise when synovial fluid collects and forms a swelling. The exact cause is unknown but risk factors include ageing and injury.

General Signs and Symptoms: Smooth, soft lump under the skin. They commonly appear on the wrist, hand and fingers, but can occur around any joint or tendon in the body. They do not tend to cause pain, but a ganglion can cause discomfort if it affects a nerve or gets particularly large.

Conventional Medical Treatment: Treatment is only usually necessary if the ganglion is causing pain or is unsightly. If this is the case, it can be removed by draining out the fluid with a needle or syringe or by surgery.

Prognosis: Harmless and may disappear without treatment.

Holistic Advice: The "old wives' tale" of hitting a ganglion with a heavy book to disperse its contents is not conventionally recommended!

Gangrene

Definition: Death of tissue in a particular area of the body. There are several types. We'll look at wet and dry.

Possible Causes: Dry gangrene is the most common. It is caused when the tissues become deprived of oxygen, possibly due to a blood clot. The tissue death is localised and does not spread from the affected site. Wet gangrene occurs when the oxygen supply to tissue is suddenly restricted by a wound (e.g. burn, frostbite, crush injury) and becomes infected with bacteria. The infection can spread to surrounding healthy tissues and can be fatal. Diabetics are susceptible to wet gangrene when a foot injury is suffered. Risk factors for gangrene include conditions that reduce blood flow, diabetes and smoking.

General Signs and Symptoms: The feet and legs are most commonly affected. In dry gangrene the skin at the affected area turns pale and cold, before turning from red to brown and then to black. The affected part withers and eventually drops off. This may be quite painless. Wet gangrene is very painful. The affected area swells before the tissues start to decay. The skin colour changes from red to brown and to then to black, and the tissues produce a foul smelling pus. The infection may also cause a fever.

Conventional Medical Treatment: Immediate hospitalisation is often required. The treatment aims to remove the affected tissue, treat the infection and address any underlying condition. Surgery or maggot therapy may be used to remove the dead tissue. In cases of wet gangrene, an area of surrounding living tissue will also be removed to attempt to control the spread of the infection. Antibiotics are commonly used. A variety of surgical techniques can be used to assist blood flow.

Prognosis: Potentially a life-threatening condition. The earlier it is diagnosed the better. If dry gangrene is caught early, the outlook is good. The outlook for wet gangrene is not so good due to the possible complications, including septicaemia (blood poisoning), caused by the infection.

Holistic Advice: Take regular exercise, stop smoking, ensure that the feet are well looked after, eat a well balanced diet, and lose any excess weight.

Gastroenteritis

Definition: Inflammation of the lining of the stomach and intestines.

Possible Causes: Usually caused by either a viral infection (e.g. norovirus) or a bacterial infection (e.g. E.coli and salmonella). Bacterial infections are often picked up from contaminated food or water, and there is an increased risk of this when travelling abroad. Most forms of gastroenteritis are highly infectious and are passed from stools to mouth when hygiene is poor.

General Signs and Symptoms: Symptoms rapidly develop and include diarrhoea, nausea, vomiting, stomach cramps and abdominal pain, fever and headache. The vomiting and diarrhoea can lead to dehydration. Symptoms of viral gastroenteritis tend to last 2-3 days, and bacterial gastroenteritis lasts 4-7 days.

Conventional Medical Treatment: Mild attacks usually clear up without treatment. Drink plenty of water to help avoid dehydration. Rehydration drinks can help rebalance the salt and sugar levels. Antidiarrhoeal drugs can help the diarrhoea but may prolong the presence of the infection. Anti-emetics can help reduce the vomiting. Antibiotics only tend to be prescribed in severe cases when a specific bacterium has been identified as the cause of the infection.

Prognosis: Usually harmless but the diarrhoea and vomiting can lead to dehydration, which can be serious for the very young and the elderly.

Holistic Advice: The risk of developing infectious gastroenteritis can be reduced by washing the hands regularly, particularly after going to the toilet and before eating. Practise good food hygiene to help prevent food poisoning and follow the recommended guidelines for safe eating and drinking when travelling abroad.

Genital Herpes

Definition: A viral infection that causes painful blisters on and around the genitals. It affects both men and women.

Possible Causes: Caused by the highly contagious herpes simplex virus (HSV). It is passed through skin-to-skin contact usually during sexual intercourse. There are two types of HSV, type 1 and type 2. Genital herpes is usually caused by type 2 HSV. Type 1 mainly causes cold sores on the mouth but can be transmitted from the mouth to the genitals where is may cause genital herpes. Once infected the virus can remain dormant within the nerves of the skin until an outbreak is triggered. Triggers may include illness, being run-down, stress and excess alcohol consumption. The changes in hormones during the menstrual cycle may trigger an outbreak in infected women.

General Signs and Symptoms: Symptoms may not appear for months even years after infection. If symptoms are to show soon after infection they usually do so within 4-7 days. Symptoms include painful, fluid-filled blisters on the genitals, thighs and buttocks that burst to leave ulcers, tingling burning and redness in the affected areas, pain on passing urine, headache, fever and muscle aches. Women may experience vaginal discharge and cervical blistering and ulceration. The first attack usually displays the worst symptoms. Recurrent infections tend to be shorter and less severe.

Conventional Medical Treatment: Anti-viral medicines (e.g. acyclovir) can be used to prevent the virus from multiplying, although it does not clear it from the body. Clinics specializing in sexually transmitted diseases (STDs) will be able to offer specialist help, advice and counselling. A pregnant women who has an attack just before childbirth may require a caesarian section to prevent infecting the baby. Painkillers and ointments for the blisters may help to relieve the symptoms.

Prognosis: There is no cure but the symptoms can generally be controlled by treatment. Genital herpes is often a chronic condition with frequent recurrences that decrease over time.

Holistic Advice: Prevention is better than (no) cure! Avoid having sex during an outbreak when the virus is very contagious. Always practise safe sex. Although using a condom does not always prevent infection (due to contact with other parts of the skin that may be infected) it will reduce the risk. Share information with partners but not towels or flannels.

Glandular Fever

Definition: A viral infection causing swollen lymph nodes, a sore throat and fatigue. Also called infectious mononucleosis.

Possible Causes: Most cases are caused by the Epstein-Barr virus (EBV). The virus attacks lymphocytes that are responsible for fighting infection. The lymphocytes pass the infection on to the lymph nodes, spleen and liver. Most EBV infections take place during childhood with few symptoms, but when it occurs during the teenage or adult years it may lead to full blown glandular fever. Glandular fever is contagious and is commonly spread through saliva. Once in the body the EBV virus remains there for life. Other far less common causes of the condition include the cytomegalovirus and rubella.

General Signs and Symptoms: Swollen lymph glands particularly in the neck, armpits and groin, very sore throat, fatigue, fever, tonsillitis, headache, swollen spleen, tender abdomen, skin rash and loss of appetite. Infections affecting the liver may cause jaundice and hepatitis.

Conventional Medical Treatment: There is no cure. Rest, drinking plenty of water, and taking painkillers such as paracetamol may help ease the symptoms. Gargling with salt water may help the sore throat. Antibiotics may be used to treat secondary infections only.

Prognosis: Most symptoms usually pass within 4-6 weeks. The associated fatigue can last for longer. Complications are uncommon but serious, including a ruptured spleen or a secondary infection of the lungs.

Holistic Advice: Anything that can help boost the immune system will help the condition. Remember that glandular fever is contagious, and contagious diseases are usually contraindicated to hands-on complementary healthcare therapies.

Glomerulonephritis

Definition: Inflammation of the glomeruli (the filtering units) of the kidneys. Note, nephritis literally means inflammation (-itis) of the kidney (nephr-). There are 2 main types, primary, where the condition occurs on its own, and secondary, where the inflammation occurs as a result of an underlying condition. Glomerulonephritis can be acute or chronic.

Possible Causes: The inflammation affects kidney function. Salt and excess fluid can build up in the body and kidney damage or even kidney failure can occur. The cause is not always known, but it may be a complication arising from infection. It is thought the body's antibodies (produced to fight the antigens that create the infection) and the antigens themselves, build up in the kidneys, causing them to become inflamed. For example, acute glomerulonephritis can develop after infection by the streptococci bacteria, which causes throat infections. It can also be a complication of more serious infections such as HIV, hepatitis B and C, and tuberculosis. Risk factors include having an autoimmune condition such as lupus, some types of glomerulonephritis run in families, long-term use of certain medications, and conditions that damage the kidneys such as cancer, leukaemia, diabetes, hypertension and liver disease.

General Signs and Symptoms: Blood and protein are passed in the urine. These may only be visibly noticeable when the kidneys have been severely damaged and so, in acute cases, may show up only in a urine test. In severe cases blood may be seen in the urine and the urine may appear cloudy or frothy. Other symptoms include the inability to urinate for 2-3 days, swollen feet and legs, puffy face, shortness of breath, headache, loss of appetite, vomiting, fever, pale skin and visual problems.

Conventional Medical Treatment: Treatment will depend on the cause and severity of the condition. In cases of bacterial infection, antibiotics may be used. If it is thought to be caused by an autoimmune disorder, immunosuppressants may be prescribed. Corticosteroids may be used to help reduce the inflammation. Diet and fluid intake will be regulated.

Prognosis: Acute cases tend to clear in 6-8 weeks. In some cases kidney function is reduced but does not deteriorate further, but others may develop chronic kidney failure. Hypertension, kidney disease and kidney failure are all known complications.

Holistic Advice: Reduce the amount of salt in the diet and drink less alcohol.

<u>Gout</u>

Definition: Gout, a common type of arthritis, is an intermittent constitutional disorder affecting small joints.

Possible Causes: Excess uric acid (a waste product of metabolism) in the blood causes crystals to form in the joints. Excess uric acid is caused either because too much is being produced or because it is not being excreted adequately by the kidneys. The excessive intake of food rich in purines is a significant risk factor. Purines are a type of acid that are found in foods such as red meats and seafood, and are also present in alcohol (especially beer). Gout can be familial and some medical conditions such as hypertension, psoriasis, diabetes, kidney problems, and high cholesterol levels can increase the risk of it developing. Some medications can also increase uric acid levels and so increase the likelihood of gout.

General Signs and Symptoms: Pain and inflammation of a joint, normally the big toe. The skin over the affected area may appear red and shiny, and may become itchy and flaky. Gout is more predominant in males over forty years old. It can attack quickly and without warning, often during the night.

Conventional Medical Treatment: Anti-inflammatory drugs are used to reduce the inflammation and the pain or, in more severe cases, corticosteroids. To prevent further attacks, drugs can be prescribed to reduce uric acid levels. Lifestyle changes to control diet, reduce alcohol intake, increase water intake, and avoid excessive weight gain are very important.

Prognosis: Gout can disappear on its own within 3-10 days. A combination of medical treatment and lifestyle changes can enable uric acid levels to be reduced, and so help prevent further attacks.

Holistic Advice: Look at diet. Avoid purine-high foods and alcohol. Try to avoid knocking the affected joint, elevate it, and keep it cool. Drink plenty of water. Uric acid levels are often higher in those who are overweight, so try to lose excess weight.

Haemorrhoids

Definition: Swollen veins inside the rectum and around the anus. Commonly called piles. There are two main types; internal (occurring inside the rectum) and external (occurring outside the rectum). Internal are more common.

Possible Causes: An increase in pressure on the blood vessels causes them to swell. This is usually as a result of straining when passing a stool. Risk factors include obesity, constipation, low-fibre diet, prolonged diarrhoea, heavy lifting, pregnancy, age and family history.

General Signs and Symptoms: Discomfort when passing a stool, bleeding from the anus after a bowel movement, discharge of mucus after a bowel movement, itchy and sore anus, and feeling that the bowels have not fully emptied. Haemorrhoids may be seen protruding from the anus. These are called prolapsed haemorrhoids.

Conventional Medical Treatment: Small haemorrhoids do not usually require treatment and clear up of their own accord. Over-the-counter creams, ointments and suppositories are available to help the itching and pain. Topical corticosteroids may be prescribed. Laxatives may ease the passing of stools in cases where the haemorrhoids are caused by constipation. Several surgical options are available, including banding (to shrink the haemorrhoid until it eventually drops off), injections (to relieve pain and destroy the haemorrhoid), infrared coagulation (to destroy the haemorrhoid using heat), or their complete surgical removal.

Prognosis: Not usually serious.

Holistic Advice: Eat a high-fibre diet. Any bleeding from the anus should be investigated by a Doctor, because it can also be indicative of a more serious disorder.

Hay Fever

Definition: Inflammation of the membrane lining the nose and throat due to an allergic reaction. Also called seasonal allergic rhinitis (inflammation of the nose).

Possible Causes: Allergic reaction to substances such as pollen or spores resulting in the inflammation of the nose, sinuses, throat and eyes. The presence of the allergen causes the cells to release histamine, which triggers the allergic reaction so causing the symptoms. Risk factors include family history or allergies, particularly asthma or eczema.

General Signs and Symptoms: Itchy eyes, throat, mouth, nose and ears, headache, violent sneezing, watery eyes and nose, and a dry cough. Usually occurs in the spring and summer when there is more pollen in the air. The severity of the hay fever depends on weather conditions and the pollen count.

Conventional Medical Treatment: Antihistamine tablets and nasal sprays help block the action of the histamine. Corticosteroid nasal spray and drops have an anti-inflammatory effect. Nasal decongestants can help blocked noses, and eye drops can help treat red, itchy eyes. Immunotherapy may be used.

Prognosis: There is no cure but the treatments can help to alleviate the symptoms. Hay fever can worsen respiratory conditions such as asthma.

Holistic Advice: Try to avoid the trigger. Avoid dairy products as these may cause additional mucus to form which can worsen the condition. Homeopathy, acupuncture and herbal remedies claim to be of benefit.

Headache (Tension)

Definition: Pain or discomfort, of variable intensity, in the head and neck.

Possible Causes: Most headaches have no underlying medical condition but are triggered by a range of factors such as stress, tension, depression, anxiety, loud noise, poor posture, bright sunlight, eyestrain, tiredness, certain foods, hunger, anger, hormonal changes, certain smells, changes in the weather and the long term use of painkillers. These are called primary headaches and include tension headaches, cluster headaches (very painful, short lived headaches that occur several times a day) and migraines (intense headache, often associated with visual disturbances and nausea). Secondary headaches are caused by an underlying condition such as meningitis and brain tumours. We'll focus on tension headaches here.

General Signs and Symptoms: Constant ache, affecting both sides of the head, tightening of neck muscles and a feeling of pressure behind the eyes. Normally comes on gradually and builds up during the day.

Conventional Medical Treatment: Over-the-counter painkillers (e.g. paracetamol) and anti-inflammatory drugs (e.g. ibuprofen) can usually relieve the pain.

Prognosis: Very common condition, generally successfully relieved by medication and changes in lifestyle.

Holistic Advice: Take measures to reduce stress, take regular exercise, practice relaxation techniques such as yoga and meditation, and reduce alcohol and caffeine intake. Medical advice should be sought if a severe headache does not respond to treatment and lasts for more than 24 hours.

Heart Attack

Definition: Sudden loss of blood supply to part of the heart muscle. The medical term for this is myocardial infarction and it is also commonly called a coronary.

Possible Causes: Usually caused by coronary artery disease. This causes the coronary arteries to narrow due to atherosclerosis. Blood clots form in the narrowed arteries and if the artery blocks completely a heart attack results. Risk factors include smoking, obesity, lack of physical activity, high fat diet, family history of coronary heart disease, hypertension and diabetes.

General Signs and Symptoms: Sudden onset of severe, crushing pain in the centre of the chest. This may spread up to the neck and into the arms, especially the left arm. The skin becomes pale and there is sweating and shortness of breath. There may be nausea and vomiting. Great anxiety, sometimes accompanied by the fear of dying, is often experienced. Contrary to popular belief, heart attacks can occur without chest pain. Always take into account the whole picture. Should the blood supply not be restored quickly the heart muscle may suffer irreversible damage and the heart may stop beating. This is called a cardiac arrest.

Conventional Medical Treatment: The priority is to relieve pain and restore the blood supply to the heart muscle. Morphine may be used for the pain and medication such as thrombolytics (to reduce the clot) and anticoagulants (to help prevent further clots) may be used. There are several surgical procedures to aid blood flow to the heart, e.g. coronary artery bypass graft (to bypass the blockage) and angioplasty (to widen the artery at the site of the blockage). The treatment usually also requires lifestyle changes. Medication such as ACE inhibitors, beta-blockers, statins and anti-platelets may be prescribed to help reduce the risk of another heart attack.

Prognosis: All heart attacks are potentially life threatening. Just over half of those who have a heart attack die but, in cases where there is not a history of heart attacks, the prognosis is good if treated quickly and there are no complications.

Holistic Advice: Treat any suspected heart attack as a medical emergency. Post-heart attack the patient may be very fearful of returning to normal activity so consider the emotional state. Eat a low fat diet. Stop smoking and reduce alcohol intake. Take regular, gentle exercise. Try to tackle any sources of stress.

Heartburn

Definition: Regurgitation of acidic stomach juices into the oesophagus. Also called Gastro-oesophageal reflex disease (GORD).

Possible Causes: Sometimes there is no obvious cause for GORD. However, it can be caused by a malfunction of the lower oesophageal sphincter, which allows stomach acid to pass back into the oesophagus. Other causes are an increased pressure on the stomach causing the reflux, and stomach acid taking longer than usual to dispel. Risk factors include being overweight, a high fat diet, tobacco, alcohol, coffee, chocolate, stress, pregnancy and the presence of a hiatus hernia.

General Signs and Symptoms: A burning sensation rising from the stomach or lower chest into the throat, and regurgitation of acid into the throat or mouth. Sufferers may also belch. Symptoms are usually worse after a large meal, at night and when lying flat. Persistent GORD can cause permanent damage and scarring to the oesophageal lining. This can lead to complications such as oesophageal ulcers, oesophageal stricture and a condition called Barrett's oesophagus in which parts of the oesophageal lining is replaced by stomach lining. Sufferers of Barrett's oesophagus have an increased risk of oesophageal cancer.

Conventional Medical Treatment: Symptoms can be relieved by making lifestyle changes and antacids are usually successful in relieving mild symptoms. If the GORD persists, treatments may be used to reduce the amount of acid produced by the stomach or increase the speed at which the stomach empties.

Prognosis: Lifestyle changes can make a difference and treatments tend to be successful. Persistent GORD has complications as described above.

Holistic Advice: Eat smaller meals, do not exercise or lie down immediately after a meal, lose excess weight and stop smoking. Avoid spicy, acidic and high fat foods, carbonated drinks, alcohol and coffee. Look for triggers that make the GORD worse and then avoid them.

<u>Heel Fissures</u>

Definition: Cracked, split heels.

Possible Causes: The fissures (cracks) are usually caused by dry skin but other causes include inactive sweat glands, prolonged standing, obesity, foot problems including heel spurs and gait. Other skin conditions such as psoriasis and eczema may increase the chance of fissures.

General Signs and Symptoms: The fissures are usually in an area of dry, callused skin. Commonly they are only superficial but if they are deep they may cause bleeding and pain which is worsened by walking. Fissures may occur on other parts of the foot, particularly the bottom of the toes.

Conventional Medical Treatment: Heel fissures are usually a cosmetic problem, not a medical one, although treatment may be necessary in extreme cases if they become infected or if any of the hard skin needs to be removed by a Doctor or Chiropodist/Podiatrist. Special foot creams can be used to help this condition. The hard skin can be gradually removed by soaking the feet in warm water and then gently rubbing them with a pumice stone. A Podiatrist may recommend insoles to correct gait or heel-cups to support the heel.

Prognosis: No permanent damage should be caused.

Holistic Advice: Buy shoes with a good shock-absorbing sole and avoid those with open-backs. Keep the feet moisturised and try to avoid the formation of calluses.

Hepatitis

Description: Inflammation of the liver, usually caused by a virus. Sometimes, in mild cases, it is asymptomatic and the person may not even be aware that they are infected and successfully fight off the virus. In others, hepatitis can cause irreversible liver damage. The condition can be acute, causing discomfort in the upper right side of the abdomen, nausea, vomiting and a fever, or chronic, causing loss of appetite, weight loss, tiredness, jaundice, swelling of the abdomen and abdominal discomfort. Cirrhosis of the liver can be caused by long-term inflammation. There are several types of hepatitis including:

Hepatitis A: Caused by the hepatitis A virus. Most common in countries with poor sanitation and sewage. It is contracted from the stools of an infected person and can be passed to others in contaminated food or water. It is usually acute and vaccinations are available.

Hepatitis B: Caused by the hepatitis B virus. The virus lives in the body fluids (e.g. blood, saliva and semen) of an infected person and is passed from person to person by direct contact with these fluids, for example during sex or sharing contaminated intravenous needles. It can be transmitted from mother to baby. Many will not even know they are infected and will successfully fight the infection but, in some, it can develop into a chronic condition. There is a vaccine available.

Hepatitis C: Caused by the hepatitis C virus. The virus is mostly found in blood but can also be found in other body fluids. It is therefore predominantly passed by blood-to-blood contact, most commonly by sharing intravenous needles. Some can fight off the infection but others may develop a chronic illness resulting in cirrhosis of the liver, even liver failure. There is no vaccine. Some drugs are available that have been shown to clear the infection in about 50% of cases.

Noninfectious Hepatitis: Inflammation of the liver can also be caused by excessive alcohol consumption, other toxins (such as those found in some poisonous fungi), some drugs, and an overdose of paracetamol. There is also an autoimmune disease, called autoimmune hepatitis, in which the white blood cells attack the liver causing severe inflammation and liver damage.

Holistic Advice: Prevention is better than cure. Practise safe sex, maintain good hand hygiene and drink alcohol responsibly. Eat a healthy, balanced diet and take regular exercise to help keep the immune system in good shape.

Hiatus Hernia

Definition: The protrusion of a portion of the stomach through the diaphragm. The general term "hernia" is used to describe the protrusion of a part of an organ through a weakened muscle. "Hiatus" is the opening in the diaphragm through which the oesophagus passes. The hiatus is the weakened area through which the stomach protrudes in a hiatus hernia.

Possible Causes: Exact cause is unknown but it may be caused by pressure on the abdomen (e.g. sudden exertion, straining, coughing and being obese), a weakened diaphragm or a congenital defect of the diaphragm. Risk factors include being female, being over 50, pregnancy, being overweight and smoking.

General Signs and Symptoms: Can be asymptomatic. However, the protrusion of the stomach through the diaphragm can prevent the sphincter at the top of the stomach from working effectively. This may allow stomach contents to pass back up into the oesophagus causing heartburn, gastro-oesophageal reflux, deep burning chest pain and difficultly swallowing.

Conventional Medical Treatment: When no symptoms are present, no treatment is required. Antacids and a change of lifestyle are recommended to begin with. A variety of drugs to counter the impact of the ineffective sphincter are available. If medication is not successful, corrective surgery can be used to return the stomach to its correct location.

Prognosis: Not usually serious but persistent acid reflux can damage the oesophagus, increasing the risk of oesophageal cancer. Rarely the hernia may become strangulated, cutting off the blood supply. This requires emergency surgery.

Holistic Advice: Lose excess weight and stop smoking. Always use correct lifting techniques when moving heavy weights.

<u>High Cholesterol</u>

Definition: Raised level of cholesterol in the blood. Called hypercholesterolaemia.

Possible Causes: Cholesterol is a lipid. It is transported around the body in the form of two types of lipoproteins, low-density (LDP) and high density (HDP). Too much LDP can cause a build up of deposits on the artery walls and so is known as "bad" cholesterol. HDP helps to carry the cholesterol back to the liver and is therefore referred to as "good" cholesterol. Blood tests are used to measure the cholesterol level and the government recommends that cholesterol levels should be less than 5mmol/L. High cholesterol levels are believed to be caused by a combination of genetic and lifestyle factors. A diet high in saturated fats, being overweight and a lack of exercise are thought to contribute. Other risk factors include smoking, diabetes, hypertension, hypothyroidism, excessive alcohol consumption, age, ethnicity, and a family history of cardiovascular disease or high cholesterol levels.

General Signs and Symptoms: High cholesterol is not a disease in itself but does increase the risk of serious cardiovascular conditions. A high cholesterol level usually goes unnoticed until it leads to the development of a disorder such as atherosclerosis. The symptoms will then be dependent on the location of the arterial narrowing.

Conventional Medical Treatment: A diet low in saturated fat can reduce levels of LDP. For those with high risk factors, making it more likely that the high cholesterol level will cause cardiovascular diseases, a change in diet is not sufficient to lower the risk, and so medication will usually be prescribed. The most common type of medication to lower cholesterol levels is statins. Other medication can be given to help reduce the risk of associated strokes and heart attacks (e.g. aspirin to help prevent blood clotting).

Prognosis: Medication and lifestyle changes tend to be successful in bringing down cholesterol levels. The extent of the risk of having a high cholesterol level depends upon the presence of risk factors. It is widely accepted that a high cholesterol level increases the risk of cardiovascular disease.

Holistic Advice: Lifestyle changes are necessary. Consult a dietician for detailed advice. Stop smoking, lose any excess weight and take regular exercise.

HIV and AIDS

Definition: A long term infection which, if left untreated, results in reduced immunity to other infections.

Possible Causes: The condition is caused by the Human Immunodeficiency Virus (HIV). HIV is spread by the exchange of body fluids including blood, semen, vagina secretions, saliva and breast milk. Transmission commonly takes place during sexual intercourse, the sharing of needles and during pregnancy when the foetus becomes infected due to the vascular connection with the mother. HIV attacks the immune system leaving the sufferer with a high risk of developing a serious infection or disease. AIDS (Acquired Immune Deficiency Syndrome) occurs when the HIV infection renders the immune system inactive and the sufferer develops a life-threatening condition such as pneumonia. AIDS now tends to be referred to as advanced or late-stage HIV infection.

General Signs and Symptoms: The initial signs of HIV infection include a fever, sore throat, tiredness, joint and muscle pain, swollen glands and a blotchy rash on the chest. After the initial symptoms, HIV may not display any symptoms for many years but will be progressively damaging the immune system. Left untreated the infection may cause a range of late-stage symptoms including persistent tiredness, night sweats, weight loss, diarrhoea, blurred vision, white spots on the tongue or mouth, dry cough, shortness of breath, fever and swollen glands. AIDS-related illnesses such as tuberculosis, pneumonia, nervous system disorders and some cancers may be caused.

Conventional Medical Treatment: There is no cure and no vaccine to stop infection, but treatments can help control the HIV infection so holding off AIDS. Highly active antiretroviral therapy (HAAT) can be successful in slowing the progression of the disease. Post Exposure Prophylaxis (PEP) may possibly halt the development of HIV if used within 72 hours of exposure to the virus.

Prognosis: The advances in treatment have transformed the prognosis from rapidly fatal condition to a long-term illness.

Holistic Advice: Prevention is the best cure. Using condoms and avoiding sex with multiple partners reduces the risk of transmission during sexual intercourse. Sufferers should make others who may come into contact with their body fluids (e.g. medical staff and dentists) aware of the infection so suitable precautions can be taken. Anything to boost the immune system may be of benefit. Emotional support and practical advice can be obtained through help groups.

Hydronephrosis

Definition: The stretching or swelling of one or both kidneys.

Possible Causes: The most common cause is a blockage in the urinary system. The blockage can be in the ureters, the point at which the renal pelvis of the kidney joins the ureter, in the bladder or in the urethra. Blockages in the ureters affect just one kidney (unilateral hydronephrosis) but blockages in the bladder and urethra affect them both (bilateral hydronephrosis). Narrowing or blocking of the ureters can be caused by many factors including an abnormality that is present at birth, a kidney stone in the ureter, growths, tumours, narrowing resulting from injury, infection, constriction, surgery, or a disorder of the nerves and muscles in the ureter. Bladder blockages can be caused by a bladder stone, blood clot, tumour, inflammation or having pressure exerted upon it (e.g. as in prostatitis). Urethral blockages can be caused by strictures and pressure. Bilateral hydronephrosis can also be caused by the backflow of urine from the bladder to the kidneys. This is usually due to a malfunction of the one-way valve in the bladder.

General Signs and Symptoms: The symptoms will depend on the location of the blockage, whether it suddenly or progressively develops, the length of time the flow of urine is interrupted, and the extent that the kidney(s) is stretched. When a blockage occurs suddenly, causing acute hydronephrosis, common symptoms include severe pain in the back or side(s), swelling in the abdomen, fever, nausea, vomiting, urinary tract infection, need to urinate frequently and painful urination. Chronic hydronephrosis can share the symptoms of the acute disease, but typically it has no symptoms or just an intermittent dull ache in the side. In such cases, chronic kidney failure may be the first sign that the condition exists.

Conventional Medical Treatment: The treatment aims to remove the build up of urine to relieve the pressure on the kidney and treat the cause of the blockage to prevent permanent kidney damage. Catheters can be inserted either into the bladder or the kidney to remove urine, and most blockages require surgery to remove them.

Prognosis: Most make a full recovery. Left untreated it can cause kidney damage or kidney failure.

Holistic Advice: Seek medical attention.

Hyperhidrosis

Definition: Excessive sweating in specific areas (focal hyperhidrosis), typically the feet, armpits, hands and face, or all over the body (generalised hyperhidrosis).

Possible Causes: Can either have no known cause (primary idiopathic hyperhidrosis) or can be symptomatic of an underlying medical condition (secondary hyperhidrosis). Most cases of focal hyperhidrosis are primary idiopathic, whilst the generalised form is usually secondary. It is thought that there is a familial link for primary idiopathic hyperhidrosis and growing evidence to suggest that it may be caused by problems with the sympathetic nervous system. Conditions that can cause secondary hyperhidrosis include hyperthyroidism, pregnancy, anxiety, substance or alcohol abuse, heart disease, respiratory failure, obesity, gout, certain infections, some types of cancer and some neurological conditions. Certain medications, including antidepressants, can also be a trigger.

General Signs and Symptoms: Excessive sweating often accompanied by an unpleasant odour. Primary idiopathic hyperhidrosis usually first appears at puberty.

Conventional Medical Treatment: Secondary (generalised) hyperhidrosis is tackled by treating the underlying condition. There are a variety of treatments for primary (focal) hyperhidrosis including lifestyle changes to improve the symptoms (e.g. avoiding known triggers, wearing antiperspirant and buying clothes made of natural fibres), prescribed antiperspirants containing aluminium chloride (to reduce the activity of the sweat glands), iontophoresis (uses an electric current to block the sweat glands) and injections of botulinum toxin may be advised in some severe cases (but the results are not permanent). If all else fails, minor operations may be performed to destroy the nerve centres that control the sweating.

Prognosis: This condition itself is not considered that serious but it is often accompanied by embarrassment and can cause emotional and psychological distress. The range of treatments is usually effective in controlling the symptoms.

Holistic Advice: Wash regularly and wear loose clothing made from natural fibres. If anxiety is a trigger, relaxation techniques may help.

Hypertension

Definition: Persistent high blood pressure (in excess of 140/90mmHg) that may damage the arteries or heart.

Possible Causes: In about 9/10 cases there is no identifiable cause but lifestyle and genetic factors are thought to contribute. Risk factors include age, family history, ethnicity, high fat diet, salt intake, lack of exercise, being overweight, smoking, excessive alcohol consumption and stress. When there is no identifiable cause it is called primary high blood pressure. In other cases the hypertension is caused by an underlying condition. This is called secondary high blood pressure. Underlying conditions that can cause hypertension include kidney conditions, atherosclerosis, some hormonal conditions (e.g. Cushing's syndrome), lupus, some medications (e.g. oral contraceptive pill and nonsteroidal anti-inflammatories) and some recreational drugs.

General Signs and Symptoms: Although usually without symptoms, very high blood pressure can cause headaches, dizziness, blurred vision, tinnitus, shortness of breath and nosebleeds.

Conventional Medical Treatment: Lifestyle changes should be made and, according to the severity of the hypertension and the presence of risk factors, antihypertensive medication may be prescribed. Common blood pressure medications include ACE inhibitors, alpha-blockers, calcium channel blockers, diuretics and beta-blockers.

Prognosis: Hypertension can damage the arteries, heart and kidneys, and is a major risk factor for developing cardiovascular disease. For most, however, medication and lifestyle changes can control the blood pressure and reduce the risk of complications.

Holistic Advice: Reduce intake of saturated fats, salt, tea, coffee and alcohol. Regular exercise, meditation and yoga can be very beneficial. Reduce any excess weight and stop smoking.

Hyperthyroidism

Definition: Overproduction of thyroid hormones. Also called thyrotoxicosis. It is one of the most common hormonal disorders.

Possible Causes: Excess thyroid hormones cause many of the body's functions to speed up. It is commonly caused by Graves' disease. Graves' disease is an autoimmune disorder in which the antibodies attack the thyroid gland, resulting in the overproduction of hormones. It can also be caused by the formation of nodules in the thyroid that increase its hormonal production. Risk factors include family history, excessive iodine in diet, other autoimmune disorders (especially vitiligo (skin condition) and pernicious anaemia, and smoking. Thyroiditis can cause acute attacks.

General Signs and Symptoms: Hyperactivity, sudden weight loss or gain, rapid heartbeat, hand tremors, excessive sweating, intolerance to heat, anxiety, insomnia, frequent bowel movements, swelling in the neck caused by an enlarged thyroid (this is called goitre), and muscle weakness. Those with Graves' disease may also have bulging eyes.

Conventional Medical Treatment: Treatment aims to reduce the amount of thyroid hormones produced. Options include antithyroid drugs, to suppress the production of the thyroid hormones, radioactive iodine, to destroy part of the thyroid, and surgical removal of a part of the thyroid or all of it. Betablockers may be prescribed to counter some of the symptoms such as the hyperactivity, rapid heartbeat and tremors.

Prognosis: Most fully recover. Some treatments may result in the thyroid producing too little thyroid hormones and so hormone supplements may be required. In very rare cases, failure to treat an overactive thyroid may result in a thyroid storm. This is a serious condition that requires urgent medical attention.

Holistic Advice: Thyroid levels should be monitored regularly after treatment. Relaxation techniques may be useful to ease hyperactivity.

Hypotension

Definition: Lower than normal blood pressure.

Possible Causes: Some people naturally have a lower than normal blood pressure and function without any problem. In other cases blood pressure may be reduced for many reasons including the side effect of some medications, heart disease, heart attack, abnormal widening of the blood vessels, serious injury, shock, autonomic disorders (e.g. diabetes mellitus, Parkinson's disease), adrenal problems, infections of the bloodstream (e.g. septicaemia), severe allergic reaction and dehydration. A common form of hypotension is postural hypertension. In this case a fall in blood pressure is experienced when the body's position is changed by suddenly standing or sitting up.

General Signs and Symptoms: Can be asymptomatic unless the pressure is very low. Symptoms may include tiredness, palpitations, weakness, light-headedness, fainting, dizziness, blurred vision and nausea.

Conventional Medical Treatment: Only usually requires treatment if the hypotension is causing symptoms. Treatment depends upon the underlying cause. Medication is rarely prescribed for hypotension.

Prognosis: Low blood pressure, if not problematic, can be of benefit as it can help protect against the conditions associated with hypertension and lessen the risk factors associated with it.

Holistic Advice: Keep hydrated and reduce caffeine and alcohol intake (particularly at night to help avoid dehydration). Eat small, frequent meals. Stand up slowly and wearing support stockings may help.

Hypothyroidism

Definition: A low level of thyroid hormones in the blood.

Possible Causes: In cases of hypothyroidism, the thyroid gland does not produce sufficient quantities of thyroid hormones (particularly thyroxine). This dysfunction of the thyroid is often brought about by an autoimmune reaction that causes the thyroid to become inflamed (thyroiditis), but can also be a side effect of the treatment for hyperthyroidism or of thyroid cancer. Severe iodine deficiency, the reaction of the thyroid to viruses or drugs, abnormal thyroid development and a problem with the pituitary gland may also rarely cause this condition.

General Signs and Symptoms: A low level of thyroxine slows many body functions. This causes weight gain, muscle aches and extreme tiredness. Other early symptoms include cramps, sensitivity to cold, constipation, slowness in body and mind, muscle weakness, dry skin, brittle hair and nails, heavy or irregular periods and depression. It may be present from birth but is more common in the over 40's, particularly women. Symptoms have a gradual onset.

Conventional Medical Treatment: Thyroxine tablets are used to rebalance the deficiency. The amount given should be regularly monitored.

Prognosis: It is a lifelong disorder but taking thyroxine will cure the symptoms.

Holistic Advice: Exercise regularly and maintain a balance diet.

Impotence

Definition: Inability to achieve or sustain an erection. Called erectile dysfunction.

Possible Causes: Occasional impotence is normal, but persistent, long-term difficulty in achieving an erection may indicate an underlying problem. It can be caused by either a physical or psychological cause, or a combination of the two. Men who are impotent with their partners, but are able to achieve erection by masturbation or wake up with an erection, are likely to have a psychological reason for the condition, e.g. anxiety, depression, relationship difficulties or the fear of failure. If an erection is not achievable under any circumstances, the cause is more likely to be physical. Conditions that may cause impotence can be those that affect blood flow to the penis (e.g. cardiovascular disease, hypertension, high cholesterol, diabetes), those that affect the nervous system (e.g. multiple sclerosis, Parkinson's disease) and hormonal conditions such as hypogonadism (which causes low levels of testosterone), hyperthyroidism and hypothyroidism. Some anatomical conditions can also affect the penile tissue. Impotence may also be a side effect of some drugs, including certain antidepressants, diuretics and antihypertensives. Risk factors include tiredness, heavy drinking, smoking and the use of illegal drugs.

General Signs and Symptoms: The inability to get and sustain an erection sufficient for satisfactory sexual intercourse.

Conventional Medical Treatment: Treatment will depend upon the underlying cause. If impotence is due to a physical condition, successfully treating that condition is likely to help. In cases caused by psychological problems, there are various forms of psychological treatments such as psychosexual counselling that may be of benefit. A variety of drugs are available to temporarily increase the blood flow to the penis (e.g. Viagra). Blood can also be encouraged to the penis with the use of a vacuum pump. Lifestyle changes to reduce the risk factors are important and they often help reduce the symptoms. Penile implants are usually only considered for those whose impotence is caused by pelvic trauma or anatomical penile problems.

Prognosis: In many cases it can be successfully treated. It can impact on the quality of life of the sufferer and his partner.

Holistic Advice: Although it is seen as an embarrassing condition, men should be encouraged to seek medical advice rather than trying to deal with it themselves.

Indigestion

Definition: Pain or discomfort in the upper abdomen, usually after eating. Also known as dyspepsia.

Possible Causes: Stomach acid comes into contact with the sensitive lining of the digestive tract, causing irritation and inflammation. It is usually associated with eating but can also be caused by infection and the reaction to certain medications. Indigestion can also be symptomatic of another condition such as gastro-oesophageal reflux, peptic ulcers or, in rare cases, stomach cancer.

General Signs and Symptoms: Symptoms include feeling bloated, heartburn, nausea and belching. Risk factors include smoking and being overweight. May be triggered by certain foods, e.g. rich, fatty, heavily spiced food, overeating, drinking excess coffee or alcohol, eating too quickly and stress.

Conventional Medical Treatment: Changes to diet and lifestyle can often reduce attacks, and antacids are usually sufficient to relieve the symptoms. A variety of other drugs to counter stomach acidity are available. If symptoms persist, worsen or are accompanied by vomiting, loss of appetite or loss of weight, a Doctor should be consulted as these can be signs of a more serious condition. Once identified, the underlying condition can then be treated, hopefully reducing the indigestion.

Prognosis: Changes to diet and lifestyle are usually sufficient unless there is an underlying medical condition. Persistent irritation of the digestive tract by stomach acid can cause serious problems.

Holistic Advice: Eat smaller portions at regular intervals, and do not eat within 3 hours of bedtime. Reduce caffeine and alcohol intake. Keep a food diary to try to ascertain any dietary triggers. Lose any excess weight and do not smoke. If possible (and, if necessary, agreed by a Doctor) avoid medicines that are known to irritate the digestive tract (e.g. aspirin).

Influenza

Definition: Infection of the upper respiratory tract. Commonly called seasonal flu.

Possible Causes: Caused by the influenza virus. The infection is highly contagious and is spread both in airborne droplets from coughs and sneezes and by direct contact. The flu virus can mutate, producing new strains to which few will have immunity.

General Signs and Symptoms: Symptoms develop 24-48 hours after infection. Symptoms usually include fever, sweating, shivering, aching muscles, exhaustion, sneezing, runny or stuffy nose, sore throat, cough and loss of appetite.

Conventional Medical Treatment: Bed rest, plenty of fluids and painkillers such as paracetamol can relieve the symptoms in most cases. Over-the-counter cold and flu remedies are also available. Medical attention should be sought if breathing problems arise, if the fever lasts for more than a couple of days or if a rash develops.

Prognosis: Symptoms usually clear up in about 5-8 days. Can be dangerous to the elderly.

Holistic Advice: The elderly and vulnerable groups can be immunized. Ensure good hand hygiene to help avoid contracting or spreading the virus. Honey and lemon drinks can be soothing. Eat a healthy, balanced diet. Boost the immune system.

Ingrown Nail

Definition: A condition in which the edge of a nail grows into the skin.

Possible Causes: Cutting nails too short, cutting the edges of the nails, tight fitting footwear, and injury to the digit can cause this condition. If the skin is warm and moist there is more chance of ingrown nails, so excessive sweating of the feet or poor hygiene may increase the incidence. Genetic factors that influence posture, gait, or the shape of the digits and nails may also contribute.

General Signs and Symptoms: Area where the nail has pierced the skin becomes red, swollen, inflamed and may bleed. The big toe is the most likely to suffer. If left untreated the digits can become infected.

Conventional Medical Treatment: In mild cases treated early, foot baths may enable the skin to be pushed back. Alternatively the part of the nail that is growing into the digit, or the whole nail, may need to be surgically removed. Painkillers may be required for the pain and antibiotics to clear any infection.

Prognosis: Very painful at the time but no lasting significant consequences.

Holistic Advice: Cut nails in a straight line, not with rounded edges. Wear shoes and socks that fit. See a GP or podiatrist as soon as a problem becomes evident.

Insomnia

Definition: Regular inability to fall asleep or stay asleep.

Possible Causes: Can be caused simply by trying to sleep in a noisy environment, but it is commonly triggered by factors such as worry, anxiety, a high intake of caffeine, alcohol and nicotine, and drug abuse. Regular sleep patterns can become quickly lost, and the insomnia becomes habitual. Insomnia can be symptomatic of some conditions that cause problems at night such as asthma, hyperthyroidism, heart disease, incontinence and arthritis, and pain may also cause the person to wake up prematurely. Insomnia is also often associated with mental health problems such as depression, mood disorders, psychotic disorders, and anxiety disorders. Some medications can cause insomnia, e.g. antidepressants, drugs for hypertension, antiepileptic drugs and non-steroidal anti-inflammatories. Insomnia is more common in women and in the elderly.

General Signs and Symptoms: Inability to go to sleep or waking during the night and being unable to get back to sleep. It can be a distressing and frustrating condition, leading to excessive tiredness, irritability and a general inability to cope. It can lead to a greater risk of accidents.

Conventional Medical Treatment: The triggers need to be tackled. Changes in lifestyle, such as taking more exercise and drinking less alcohol and caffeine, can be of benefit. Guidance will be given on how to promote good sleeping patterns, such as keeping regular bedtimes, avoiding food late at night and trying to relax before bedtime. Sleeping tablets can be used short-term to help restore the sleeping pattern but should not be taken long-term. Cognitive and behavioral treatments may be of use to change thoughts and behaviour patterns that may be worsening the problem.

Prognosis: If caused by an underlying medical condition, then treating that will often help. Tackling any worries or anxieties, making life style changes and creating a bedtime routine will usually help the insomnia to disappear.

Holistic Advice: Ensure the bedroom is a relaxing, calm environment that is conducive to sleep. Avoid watching television or using electric equipment such as mobile phones and computers just before bedtime, and try not to have them in the bedroom. Develop a bedtime routine. Take regular exercise, eat a balanced, healthy diet and avoid alcohol, caffeine and spicy foods (particularly just before bedtime). Give up smoking.

Irritable Bowel Syndrome

Definition: Chronic condition of the digestive system causing intermittent abdominal pain, diarrhoea and constipation. Abbreviated to IBS.

Possible Causes: The exact cause of IBS is not know but possible physical and psychological contributing factors include the abnormal contraction of the muscles in the intestinal walls, sensitivity of the digestive organs to pain, immune system problems, problems with how the central nervous system controls the digestive system, an unusual response to infection, sensitivity to certain foods, environmental and genetic factors, stress and depression.

General Signs and Symptoms: Common symptoms can include abdominal pain, changes in bowel habits, bloating and swelling of the abdomen, a feeling of fullness and difficulty in finishing meals, excessive wind, nausea and vomiting, an urgent need to defaecate, feeling that the bowel has not fully emptied after defaecation and the passing of mucus from the rectum. Symptoms are usually worse after eating and can fluctuate in severity, with periods of remission and relapse. Other symptoms may include lower back pain, muscle and joint pain, constant tiredness, headache, belching, halitosis and a frequent and urgent need to urinate. IBS is twice as common in women then men and normally develops between the ages of 20-30 but can affect any age.

Conventional Medical Treatment: There is no cure but the symptoms can often be controlled by a combination of lifestyle and dietary changes and relaxation techniques. If symptoms persist medication may be required to treat the symptoms. Antispasmodic medicines (to reduce abdominal pain and cramping), laxatives (to combat constipation), antimotility medicines (to treat diarrhoea) and tricyclic antidepressants (to reduce abdominal pain and cramping) may be prescribed. Psychological therapies may also be used to help control the condition.

Prognosis: IBS poses no serious threat to health, but there is a need to rule out other more serious digestive disorders which display similar symptoms.

Holistic Advice: Keep a food diary to try to identify any dietary triggers. Eat regularly, drink plenty of water and reduce alcohol and coffee consumption. Probiotics may help. Exercise regularly to keep fit and defuse stress. Anything that reduces stress, such as relaxation techniques and yoga, may help. Acupuncture, reflexology and aloe vera (a herbal remedy) may be of benefit.

Jaundice

Definition: Yellow discoloration of the skin and the whites of the eyes. It is a symptom of disease, not a condition itself.

Possible Causes: Jaundice results from excessively high levels of a yellowish pigment called bilirubin in the blood. Bilirubin originates in the red blood cells. The liver breaks down bilirubin and excretes it. If for any reason the liver cannot remove the bilirubin, jaundice occurs. There are 3 main reasons for jaundice - 1. In hepatocellular jaundice, the liver is damaged and unable to process the bilirubin. 2. In haemolytic jaundice, too many red blood cells are broken down so the liver can't cope with the quantity of bilirubin in the blood. 3. In obstructive jaundice, the bile duct is blocked, causing a backlog of bilirubin in the liver which is forced back into the blood. Jaundice can be a symptom of many disorders of the liver, gall bladder, and pancreas. It may also be caused by some blood disorders. Jaundice is common in a newly born baby if the liver is not fully functional. This usually resolves in about a week.

General Signs and Symptoms: Yellow discoloration of the skin and the whites of the eyes. The body fluids may also appear discoloured. Depending on the cause of the jaundice, symptoms may also include tiredness, abdominal pain, itchy skin, vomiting, weight loss and fever.

Conventional Medical Treatment: Investigation is always required to establish the underlying medical condition that is causing the jaundice. If the underlying condition can be treated, the jaundice will disappear.

Prognosis: Depends upon the underlying condition.

Holistic Advice: Take measures to keep the liver healthy, such as drinking plenty of fluids, reducing alcohol intake, maintaining a healthy, balanced diet, and taking regular exercise.

Kidney Stones

Definition: Crystallized deposits that build up in the one or both of the kidneys. Also called nephrolithiasis.

Possible Causes: Crystallization of waste products in the kidney which, over time, build up into a hard stone. They are usually formed following a build up of calcium (the most common type), ammonia, uric acid or cystine. The exact cause is unknown but risk factors include insufficient fluid intake, immobility, family history, repeated urinary infections, history of kidney stones, only having one kidney and diseases of the small intestine. Medications such as aspirin, antacids, and calcium and vitamin D supplements can also increase the risk, as does the treatment used for certain medical conditions such as cancer or kidney disease.

General Signs and Symptoms: Small stones often pass unnoticed. Symptoms only tend to be caused if the stone gets stuck in the kidney, when it travels down the ureter, or if it causes an infection. Symptoms of kidney stones are collectively referred to as renal colic and include severe pain in the back or side of the abdomen, restlessness, nausea, vomiting, blood in the urine, cloudy or smelly urine, burning sensation on urination, fever and a feeling that urination is necessary even if it is not. If the stone is passed in the urine the pain rapidly subsides. However, if they get stuck hydronephrosis and kidney infections can be caused.

Conventional Medical Treatment: The treatment depends on the stone. Small stones may just pass in the urine and medication can be taken to relieve the pain, nausea and vomiting. Large stones may need treatment to remove them. The most common treatment is lithotripsy, which involves sending high-energy shock waves through the stone to break it up. Percutaneous nephrolithotomy is a technique in which a nephroscope is passed into the kidney to remove the stone. Ureterorenoscopy techniques can be used to remove a stone from a ureter. For large stones conventional surgery is sometimes required.

Prognosis: Complications are rare but kidney stones often recur.

Holistic Advice: Those prone to stones should drink up 2-3 litres of fluid a day, especially during hot weather or when perspiring. Dehydration will increase the concentration of the urine, so increasing the risk of kidney stones and disorders such as cystitis. Empty the bladder as soon as you need to because the longer the urine remains in the body, the more likely it is that the minerals will crystallize. Dietary changes may help according to the type of stone.

Laryngitis

Definition: Inflammation of the larynx.

Possible Causes: Acute laryngitis is usually caused by a viral Infection (e.g. the common cold or flu) or physical injury (caused by shouting, prolonged singing or by swallowing very hot fluids). Chronic laryngitis can be caused by smoking, alcohol misuse, gastro-oesophageal reflux, and a range of environmental factors (e.g. long term exposure to dust, fumes and chemicals). Dry air from central heating can aggravate the condition.

General Signs and Symptoms: The larynx appears red and swollen. This is accompanied by hoarseness or a complete loss of the voice, sore painful throat, mild fever, a loud, barking, rough or husky cough, and a constant need to clear the throat. Inspiration and expiration can be difficult, particularly in children.

Conventional Medical Treatment: Acute laryngitis has no medical treatment as such. Resting the vocal cords, keeping hydrated and boosting the immune system are recommended. Antibiotics will only be given if there is a bacterial infection. Chronic laryngitis is treated according to its cause. Mostly this will involve lifestyle changes.

Prognosis: Most sufferers of acute laryngitis will make a full recovery without any complications. Chronic laryngitis takes longer to clear and can cause permanent damage.

Holistic Advice: Rest the voice. If laryngitis is due to an infection following a cold, cough or sore throat, then look at boosting the immune system. Steam inhalation may be of benefit. Stop smoking, avoid smoky environments and reduce alcohol intake. Laryngitis can cause great frustration as well as discomfort, so treat the whole person.

Leg Ulcer

Definition: A persistent open sore, usually on the lower part of the leg.

Possible Causes: Leg ulcers commonly occur when the skin breaks down due to poor circulation. An open sore then develops, either spontaneously or following a minor injury. There are several types of leg ulcer: venous – occur on the veins, arterial – occur on the arteries, diabetic – occur due to high blood sugar associated with diabetes, vasculitic – due to chronic inflammatory disorders, traumatic – caused by injury, and malignant – caused by a skin tumour. Venous leg ulcers are the most common. Risk factors include compromised circulation, age, immobility, diabetes, obesity, deep vein thrombosis and varicose veins.

General Signs and Symptoms: Initially there is pain, itching and swelling on the affected leg. The skin breaks and the ulcer appears as a shallow, pink area of broken skin. The surrounding tissue may be swollen. They are often painful and very slow to heal.

Conventional Medical Treatment: The ulcers are cleaned and dressed. Compression bandages may be used to help control the blood pressure in the legs. The underlying reason for the ulcer will be addressed. If the ulcer becomes infected, antibiotics may be prescribed.

Prognosis: May take several months to heal. If circulation or immobility is not improved they may return.

Holistic Advice: Take regular exercise to improve circulation. Lose any excess weight and stop smoking. Keep the legs moisturised and inspect them regularly for signs of skin damage.

Lupus

Definition: Chronic autoimmune condition that causes inflammation in the body's tissues. There are 2 main types. The most common is systemic lupus erythematosus (SLE) which affects the whole body. Discoid lupus erythematosus only affects the skin. We'll focus on SLE here.

Possible Causes: In this autoimmune condition the body produces antibodies that react against its own connective tissues causing them to become inflamed and swollen. The exact cause is unknown but it is thought to be a combination of genetic and environmental factors. Possible triggers include viruses, infections, some medications, exposure to sunlight, hormonal changes and childbirth.

General Signs and Symptoms: The condition is characterized by intermittent flare ups of joint pain (particularly in the hands and feet), fatigue and skin rashes (commonly on the face, wrists and hands). Other possible symptoms include fever, changes in weight, swollen glands, recurring mouth ulcers, alopecia, hypertension, migraine, anaemia, Raynaud's disease (which limits the blood supply to the hands), increased sensitivity to sunlight, depression and anxiety. Symptoms vary from person to person and range from mild to severe.

Conventional Medical Treatment: Lupus may be treated with non-steroidal anti-inflammatories, hydroxychloroquine, cortiosteroids and immunosuppressants.

Prognosis: There is no cure but the treatments can usually manage the symptoms. For some sufferers, lupus can lead to more serious conditions such as kidney damage, other autoimmune conditions, blood and heart conditions, and pleurisy.

Holistic Advice: Protect the skin and eyes from the sun. Physiotherapy may be useful for joint problems.

Lymphadenopathy

Definition: Enlarged lymph nodes.

Possible Causes: Lymph nodes most commonly become swollen due to a bacterial or viral infection. The lymph nodes in the neck, groin and armpits are closer to the surface and so these are the ones that are usually noticed. The swelling will usually subside when the infection clears up. Many conditions caused by infection will have lymphadenopathy as a symptom, for example the lymph nodes in the neck commonly swell during tonsillitis. Some medical conditions can cause long term lymphadenopathy, e.g. tuberculosis and AIDS. Persistent swelling of many or all the lymph nodes may be indicative of some types of cancer such as breast cancer, lymphoma and leukaemia.

General Signs and Symptoms: Swollen and sometime painful lymph nodes. When caused by cancer, the swollen lymph nodes do not usually feel painful.

Conventional Medical Treatment: Treating the underlying cause will usually cure this condition. Antibiotics can help bacterial infections.

Prognosis: No complications unless caused by a serious underlying condition.

Holistic Advice: Boost the immune system to help the body combat the infection.

Lymphoedema

Definition: Localised accumulation of fluid in the lymphatic vessels causing swelling in the body's tissues.

Possible Causes: Lymphoedema is caused by damage or disruption to the lymphatic system which renders it unable to successfully drain fluid away from the tissues. The excess fluid accumulates in the tissues and causes the tissues to swell. There are 2 types - primary, which is caused by faulty genes and develops at birth or shortly after puberty and, more commonly, secondary, which may be caused by infection (especially cellulitis), inflammatory diseases (e.g. rheumatoid arthritis, dermatitis and eczema), cardiovascular diseases (e.g. deep vein thrombosis and venous leg ulcers), cancer of the lymphatic system, cancer treatments that cause harm to the lymphatic system, trauma and injury.

General Signs and Symptoms: Typically the swelling is in the arms or legs but other places may be affected. Limbs may feel heavy, lose mobility and be painful. There may be tingling, skin infections and skin conditions such as blisters and wart-like growths.

Conventional Medical Treatment: Manual lymphatic drainage, multilayer lymphoedema bandaging, remedial exercises and skin care combine to help treat the symptoms. Surgery may be possible in the form of liposuction to remove excess fat from the area which can reduce the swelling.

Prognosis: Lymphoedema is a life long disorder with no cure, but symptoms can usually be controlled using a combination of treatments. Any damage to the skin can quickly lead to infection and be slow to heal. Sufferers run a high risk of cellulitis which can be treated with antibiotics.

Holistic Advice: Take great care with the skin, lose excess weight and maintain a healthy diet. Avoid alcohol and spicy food as they may increase swelling. Air travel may also worsen the condition. Elevate the affected limbs when possible. Sufferers are often very aware that the condition has a negative effect on appearance and so they may be self conscious, stressed and depressed.

Mastitis

Definition: Inflammation of the breast tissue.

Possible Causes: The most common cause is milk not being completely removed from the breast during breastfeeding. It commonly occurs in the first 6 weeks of breastfeeding but it can also develop if breastfeeding is suddenly stopped and the breasts become overfilled with milk. There are 2 main types - non-infectious, which is caused by the surplus milk blocking the milk ducts, and infectious, which is caused by a bacterial infection. Left untreated non-infectious mastitis can become infectious, due to bacteria infecting the remaining milk. Mastitis can also be experienced by non-breastfeeding women and is caused by bacterial infection. It is more common in smokers and those pre and post menopause.

General Signs and Symptoms: Breast tissue becomes swollen, sore, red, hard, and may feel lumpy. It usually only affects one area of a breast. There may be flu-like symptoms with a fever and chills. There may be a discharge from the nipple.

Conventional Medical Treatment: The continuation of breast feeding will help to remove the blocked milk and improve the symptoms. Advice may be given on breastfeeding techniques. Painkillers can be taken to ease the pain and warm compresses on the affected part of the breast may give relief. Infectious mastitis may need antibiotics.

Prognosis: Left untreated the inflammation caused by infectious mastitis can worsen and a breast abscess may develop.

Holistic Advice: Take rest and drink plenty of fluids. Any breast lumps or noticeable changes in the breast tissue should be examined by a Doctor.

<u>Meningitis</u>

Definition: Inflammation of the meninges (the membranes that cover the brain and spinal cord).

Possible Causes: Most often caused by a bacterial or viral infection of the meninges. The infection causes the meninges to swell, which can lead to nerve and brain damage. Bacterial meningitis is the most serious and should be treated as a medical emergency. It is most commonly caused by the meningococcal bacteria or the streptococcus bacteria. If left untreated it can lead to serious brain damage and blood poisoning. It is spread by coughing, sneezing, sharing objects that have been in the mouth, such as cutlery, toothbrushes and cigarettes. Viral meningitis is the most common type and is often mistaken for flu. The virus (commonly enteroviruses or herpes simplex) is spread by coughing, sneezing and contact with contaminated objects. Those with a weakened immune system are at greater risk of contracting all types of meningitis.

General Signs and Symptoms: The symptoms of bacterial meningitis have a rapid onset and quickly worsen. In adults, meningitis may first show as mild fever with general aches and pains, and the skin may appear pale or blotchy. The symptoms then rapidly progress and may include severe headache, vomiting, fever, stiff neck, sensitivity to light, drowsiness, confusion and fits. There may be a distinctive reddish-purple skin rash that does not disappear when pressed. Babies may appear unresponsive and floppy or stiff and jerky, be very sleepy, adopt a staring expression, have a loss of appetite, vomit, have pale and blotchy skin, cry and be irritable but not want to be held. Most with viral meningitis show only flu-like symptoms but in severe cases a stiff neck, muscle and joint pain, nausea, vomiting, diarrhoea, and sensitivity to light may be experienced.

Conventional Medical Treatment: Intravenous antibiotics are used to treat bacterial meningitis. The patient will need to be monitored carefully and may require oxygen, fluids and steroids to reduce the inflammation. Viral meningitis is usually mild and treated at home with painkillers and anti-emetics (for the sickness). Severe cases will be treated in the same way as bacterial meningitis until it is definitely confirmed to be viral and then the antibiotics withdrawn.

Prognosis: Viral meningitis usually gets better in a few weeks. Bacterial meningitis causes death in about 10% of cases, and complications such as hearing problems are common.

Holistic Advice: Prevention is better than cure and vaccinations are available to help protect against some strains. Boost the immune system.

Menorrhagia

Definition: Heavier than normal bleeding during menstruation.

Possible Causes: Sometimes the cause is not apparent and, particularly for those who normally have heavy periods, there is probably no need for concern. However, it can be a symptom of uterine disorders such as fibroids, polyps, endometriosis, persistent pelvic infections, polycystic ovary syndrome, or cancer of the uterus, and can also be caused by hormonal disorders such as hypothyroidism. It may be a side effect of using an intrauterine contraceptive device. Risk factors include being over weight, approaching the menopause, anti-coagulant medicines and chemotherapy.

General Signs and Symptoms: Heavy menstrual bleeding which may include blood clots. There may be a dragging pain in the lower abdomen.

Conventional Medical Treatment: Depends on the cause and severity of the condition. A variety of drugs can be prescribed to reduce or stop the bleeding. Depending on the cause, surgical options may be possible. A hysterectomy will stop menstrual bleeding but is only considered as a last resort.

Prognosis: Severe menstrual bleeding, if left untreated, may lead to iron deficiency anaemia.

Holistic Advice: Can cause disruption to many aspects of life style, affecting the woman physically, emotionally and socially.

Migraine

Definition: Intense headache. There are two types – common migraine, which is a severe headache with no warning symptoms, and classical migraine, in which the headache is experienced after warning symptoms (collectively know as the "aura") such as visual disturbances, anxiety, mood swings, changes in energy levels, co-ordination problems, speech difficulties, muscular stiffness or tingling in the neck and shoulders, and an altered sense of taste and smell.

Possible Causes: Thought to be caused by chemical changes in the brain. The aura may be caused by a sudden restriction of blood flow to the brain, and the migraine itself is associated with an increased blood flow. There are many possible trigger factors including hormonal changes associated with menstruation or menopause, anxiety, stress, tension (particularly in the neck and shoulders), shock, depression, excitement, irregular meals, prolonged lack of food, diet, alcohol, over-exertion, physical and mental fatigue, changes of routine, late rising (too much sleep), some medicines, fluorescent lights, flickering screens, changes in weather and sensitivity to certain substances, e.g. paint, petrol, perfume.

General Signs and Symptoms: Commonly a throbbing pain at the front or on one side of the head, worsened by movement. The migraine itself may cause nausea and an increased sensitivity to light, sounds and smells. Body temperature may fluctuate, concentration may be affected, and there may be abdominal pain and a need to urinate frequently. In attacks of classical migraine, the aura, as described above, is experienced first. Symptoms of migraine can last from a few hours to several days and are more common in women than men.

Conventional Medical Treatment: Painkillers, anti-inflammatory drugs, and anti-sickness medicines are commonly used to ease the symptoms. More specific anti-migraine drugs, such as triptan medicines, may be prescribed. Triptan medicines, if taken at the beginning of an episode or during the aura stage, may prevent the migraine from developing further.

Prognosis: There is no cure but, although they can be disabling, migraine episodes can usually be managed by the effective use of treatments.

Holistic Advice: A regular massage can be a very good preventative treatment to release stress and tension. Keep a diary of food eaten to see if diet is the cause. Cheese, chocolate and red wine are the most common dietary triggers. Eat regularly, follow a regular sleep pattern, and try to reduce stress.

Motor Neurone Disease

Definition: Progressive degeneration of the nerves in the brain and spinal cord that control muscular activity.

Possible Causes: The motor neurones lose function but the exact cause is unknown. There may be a familial link. There are several types of motor neurone disease. They all have similar symptoms but the speed of progression varies.

General Signs and Symptoms: The motor neurones control voluntary activity such as walking, speaking, breathing and swallowing and so these functions are affected by this condition. Initially sufferers experience muscle weakness, clumsiness, general tiredness, muscle pains, cramps and twitches, and slurred speech. As the condition progresses there is muscle wastage, loss of mobility in the limbs, muscle pain, speech difficulties, drooling, excessive yawning, and problems swallowing. The condition may result in total paralysis and severe breathing difficulties. There may be mood swings and understandably the sufferer often becomes anxious and depressed.

Conventional Medical Treatment: Riluzole is the only drug that may directly help the condition but it only gives about another 3 months of life. Other treatments focus on relieving the symptoms both physical and emotional, and so counsellors, physiotherapists and speech therapists may all be involved. A plan will be put in place to ensure the care given when the sufferer can no longer communicate is what was wanted.

Prognosis: It is a rare, serious and incurable disease.

Holistic Advice: Support groups can offer advice and self-help guidance for the sufferer and his/her family.

Mouth Ulcer

Definition: An open sore on the lining of the mouth. The medical name is aphthous ulcer.

Possible Causes: Usually non-infectious and caused as a result of damage to the mouth tissues (e.g. biting the inside of the cheek or rough tooth brushing). Risk factors include stress, anxiety, hormonal changes, certain foods, family history and a depressed immune system. Recurrent mouth ulcers may occasionally be symptomatic of an underlying disease such as iron deficiency, vitamin B_{12} deficiency, folic acid deficiency and some intestinal disorders. Mouth ulcers can also occur as a result of a specific infection such as herpes simplex and pharyngitis.

General Signs and Symptoms: Shallow, grey-white pits with a red border. They can cause pain when eating spicy, hot or acidic foods. Can occur singly or in clusters.

Conventional Medical Treatment: Usually disappear without treatment in a few days. Salty mouth washes may help (don't swallow and seek advice in cases of cardiac problems). Over-the-counter treatments are available.

Prognosis: Usually harmless but consult a Doctor if they do not heal within 3 weeks.

Holistic Advice: To help speed up the healing of a mouth ulcer, use a soft toothbrush, avoid hard foods and try to reduce stress levels.

Multiple Sclerosis

Definition: A progressive disease of the brain and spinal cord in which the insulating sheaths of the nerves break up and patches of excessive connective tissue form. Abbreviated to MS.

Possible Causes: MS is an autoimmune disease. It is not known for certain what causes it, but some believe it is caused by a combination of genetic and environmental factors.

General Signs and Symptoms: This condition can have a slow onset and can remit and relapse. The progressive nerve damage affects sensation, movement, body functions and balance. The central nervous system controls the whole body and so, potentially, any part of the body could be affected, but the extent and severity of the symptoms depend on the site and progression of the disease. Numbness and tingling in the extremities commonly occur in the early stages, and in 25% of cases the first symptom is inflammation of the optic nerve, causing visual problems. General weakness and tremors are common upon exertion and sufferers may feel persistent extreme tiredness. There can be muscle spasms causing stiffness, and neuromuscular pain. Speech may become slurred. Problems with co-ordination and cognition may be experienced and it is not uncommon for sufferers to have emotional problems and depression. Stress and heat can worsen the symptoms. MS is the most common nervous system disorder affecting young adults and is twice as likely to affect women than men.

Conventional Medical Treatment: Due to the unpredictability of the condition and the variety of symptoms, care plans will vary. Specialists may be needed to assist mobility, speech, sight, continence and any psychological problems. Drugs to treat some of the symptoms include steroids, painkillers, muscle relaxant drugs, anti-tremor drugs, and antidepressants. Specialist drugs can also be injected to slow the progression of nerve damage.

Prognosis: There is no cure and it is a lifelong condition, but the treatments make it easier to live with. MS does not affect life expectancy but the nerve damage may cause partial paralysis and an affected person may ultimately require a wheelchair for mobility.

Holistic Advice: Take regular, gentle exercise. Yoga can be beneficial to help relaxation as well as stretching the muscles. Reflexology, massage, acupuncture, tai chi and other complementary therapies may help. Minimise stress and avoid high temperatures. There are many support groups for sufferers of MS and their families to get help and advice.

Muscular Dystrophy

Definition: A group of genetic conditions in which muscles become weak and wasted.

Possible Causes: All types of muscular dystrophy are caused by genetic mutations in the genes that control muscular structure and function. The mutations can occur spontaneously but they are usually inherited. Duchenne muscular dystrophy is the most common and the most severe. It affects boys and shows at about the age of 3 years. It begins in the leg muscles before quickly progressing to cause serious disability. Myotonic muscular dystrophy is the most common form in adults. It affects the smaller muscles such as the face, jaws and neck of both sexes.

General Signs and Symptoms: Symptoms vary according to the type of muscular dystrophy and the age of the person when the condition first appeared. For example, in the case of Duchenne muscular dystrophy the legs are first affected so there are problems walking and standing up. The sufferer is usually wheelchair-bound in a few years, develops a curvature (scoliosis) of the spine, has heart problems by the mid-teens, respiratory problems by the late-teens, and is likely to die before the age of 30. In myotonic muscular dystrophy there may be muscle stiffness, cataracts and hormonal problems. The condition is often slow to progress. Some may never progress to serious disability although cardiac problems are possible.

Conventional Medical Treatment: Maintaining mobility for as long as possible is important and so exercise, physiotherapy and physical aids (e.g. braces, crutches and wheelchairs) are used. Some drugs can be used to try to increase muscle strength. Scoliosis of the spine can be corrected by surgery. Cardiac problems can be treated in a variety of ways as and when they occur.

Prognosis: Muscular dystrophy is a progressive disease which becomes life threatening if the cardiac or respiratory muscles are affected. There is no cure but the treatments may help to manage the condition.

Holistic Advice: Support groups can offer advice and self-help guidance for the sufferer and his/her family.

Myalgic Encephalomyelitis

Definition: Abbreviated to M.E., it literally means muscle pain and inflammation of the brain and spinal cord. Also called chronic fatigue syndrome.

Possible Causes: The cause is uncertain, but some think it can be triggered by viral infections that weaken the immune system, e.g. glandular fever, hence it is sometimes referred to as post viral fatigue. Others believe it to be triggered by a combination of physical and psychological factors such as exhaustion, depression, traumatic events, repeated infections, inactivity (or being too active), stress, frustration and poor diet.

General Signs and Symptoms: The main characteristic is generally feeling unwell and extreme fatigue that doesn't decrease with sleep. There are many other possible symptoms including a sore throat, swollen lymph glands, stomach pain, muscle and joint pain (but without inflammation), headaches, intolerance to light, loud noise, alcohol and certain foods, giddiness, palpitations, mood swings, sleeping problems, an inability to concentrate and poor memory. Exercise may worsen the symptoms.

Conventional Medical Treatment: There is no cure, so the treatment focuses on easing the symptoms. The psychological side may be helped by cognitive behavioural therapy to identify thoughts and feelings that trigger behaviour, antidepressants, painkillers, and a tailored exercise programme.

Prognosis: May last for many years. Most cases improve over time enough to resume a normal life, but others continue having symptoms and relapses. Some remain housebound. Early diagnosis, balancing rest with activity, and self help measures can assist.

Holistic Advice: Take plenty of rest and avoid stress of any kind. Maintain a balanced diet. When feeling weak, find an activity that can still be undertaken e.g. a jigsaw. Try relaxation exercises or a massage. Exercise regularly at whatever level can be managed.

Myasthenia Gravis

Definition: Literally means grave muscle weakness. It only affects voluntary muscles.

Possible Causes: Chronic autoimmune disease in which the body produces antibodies that block or damage muscle receptor cells. This causes muscle weakness and excessive muscle fatigue. May be triggered by some viruses or medicines. Genetic make up may also have a role to play although it is not familial.

General Signs and Symptoms: Muscle weakness that gets worse as the day goes on or after activity. Most commonly affects the eye muscles (causing drooping of the eyelid), face and throat muscles (affecting smiling, speech, chewing and swallowing), neck muscles (making it difficult to support the head), and the limbs (creating problems with tasks such as walking upstairs or holding the arms above the head). More rarely, the condition may affect the respiratory muscles, making breathing difficult when exercising or when lying flat. Myasthenia gravis is not usually painful and symptoms that are mild at first get worse over several months.

Conventional Medical Treatment: Cholinesterase inhibitors, to block the action of the chemical that makes muscles relax post-contraction, removal of the thymus gland, which is commonly abnormal in patients with this condition, and steroids and immunosuppressant drugs, to reduce the number of associated antibodies produced, are used to help alleviate symptoms.

Prognosis: No cure but the symptoms can usually be controlled.

Holistic Advice: Try to reduce stress levels and over-exertion. Promote good sleeping habits. The Myasthenia Gravis Association may be able to offer valuable support.

Nail Conditions (Additional)

General Information:

Nails may change shape, colour or texture. This is may be due to injury, infection, lifestyle or an underlying disease. Some drugs may also affect the nails.

Minor nail abnormalities that are not associated with underlying disorders, such as white spots caused by minor injury, are unlikely to need treatment. However, if the shape, colour or general condition of the nails changes when no obvious damage has occurred a Doctor should be consulted.

Once the cause of the underlying condition has been treated, the nails should begin to grow normally again. A finger nail can take 6-9 months to grow out and so the process can be slow but the appearance and health of the nails may be improved by having regular manicures or help from a chiropodist.

We have already looked at onychomycosis. On the next page the following other nail conditions will be summarised:

- ➢ Blue Nails
- ➢ Discoloured Nails
- ➢ Habit Tic
- ➢ Koilonychia
- ➢ Onychogryphosis
- ➢ Pitting
- ➢ Ridged Nails
- ➢ Vertical Streaks

Nail Conditions (Additional) Continued

Discoloured Nails: Nails may become discoloured for many reasons including infection, trauma, lifestyle and an underlying medical disorder. Here are a few examples of the most common causes:
Yellow nails - infection or heavy smoking
Green nails - infection
White nails - nail damage, onycholysis or indicative of liver or kidney disease
Black nails - collection of blood under the nail from trauma or infection
Blue nails: may be symptomatic of argyria (caused by the improper exposure to compounds of silver) or Wilson's disease (in which copper builds up in the body) or a lack of oxygen in the blood

Habit Tic: The nail shows damage caused by the habitual picking, scratching or biting of the nail or surrounding tissue.

Koilonychia: Concave spoon-shaped nails. This is usually caused by severe iron deficiency.

Onychogryphosis: Thickening of the nails. May be due to trauma, neglect or fungal infection. Mostly affects toe nails.

Pitting: Multiple tiny pits show on the surface of the nail. This is often indicative of an underlying disease such as psoriasis or eczema. It may also be associated with alopecia.

Ridged Nails: The occurrence of longitudinal ridges is normal in the elderly. In younger people it may be indicative of rheumatoid arthritis, lichen planus (a skin condition) and eczema.

Vertical Streaks: Vertical streaks are also normal in the elderly and are not usually associated with any underlying disorder.

Neuralgia

Definition: Literally means nerve (neur-) pain (-algia). There are 2 main types - trigeminal neuralgia, which is a sudden and severe nerve pain that affects the face for just a few minutes, and postherpetic neuralgia, which is a constant and severe nerve pain brought on by shingles.

Possible Causes: Trigeminal neuralgia is thought to be caused by blood vessels pressing on the root of the trigeminal nerve. It may also be caused by a tumour or multiple sclerosis. Postherpetic neuralgia is caused by the shingles virus. The shingles virus damages the nerves and it is thought that the scar tissue which develops may press on the nerves causing the pain.

General Signs and Symptoms: In trigeminal neuralgia the stabbing, shooting pain is usually felt on only one side of the face, and only for a very short time. The episodes may repeat 100s of times a day or not recur for years. Pain is usually in the jaws, cheek, eye and forehead and may be felt in the mouth. The pain may be triggered by certain actions or movement. Sufferers of postherpetic neuralgia will experience a constant and severe burning, aching or throbbing where the shingles occurred, some stabbing or shooting pain and intense itching.

Conventional Medical Treatment: Anticonvulsants (to prevent seizures) can be effective for trigeminal neuralgia (normal painkillers are not strong enough). Surgery may be necessary. Painkillers, analgesic creams and antidepressants are the most common treatment for postherpetic neuralgia although anticonvulsants may also be used.

Prognosis: Trigeminal neuralgia is a chronic condition that often gets worse over time. Symptoms can be treated but surgery may be required. Postherpetic neuralgia can get better after a few months but can last much longer. Treatment may not completely relieve the pain.

Holistic Advice: For trigeminal neuralgia, avoid wind and draughts, and be wary of eating and drinking hot or cold foods. In cases of posthepetic neuralgia, wear loose fitting clothing and cover sensitive areas to prevent rubbing. Cold packs may help.

<u>Non-Specific Urethritis</u>

Definition: Inflammation of the urethra not caused by gonorrhoea.

Possible Causes: Non-specific urethritis is the term used when the cause is not known but it has been established that it is NOT caused by gonorrhoea (a sexually transmitted bacterial infection). However, a sexually transmitted disease called chlamydia, caused by the chlamydia trachomatis bacteria, is often responsible for non-specific urethritis. It can also be caused by urinary tract infections and infections from other bacteria or viruses, particularly those that live in the throat, mouth and rectum that find their way into the urethra. Non-specific urethritis can also be caused by damage to the urethra or its irritation by products it may come into contact with.

General Signs and Symptoms: Men may experience a discharge from the penis, pain on urinating, frequent need to urinate, and redness at the opening of the urethra. Mild cases may be asymptomatic. Women only tend to show symptoms if the inflammation spreads to other parts of the pelvis.

Conventional Medical Treatment: Antibiotics are commonly used to treat any bacterial infection.

Prognosis: Can usually be treated effectively but, in women, if the infection spreads it can cause pelvic inflammatory disease which is a serious and painful disorder. In men there is a danger of persistent urethritis. Sexual health clinics will be able to give advice.

Holistic Advice: Practice safe sex to help avoid contracting the condition. If infected, avoid sex altogether until the infection has cleared up completely.

Nosebleed

Definition: Bleeding from the nose. The medical term is epistaxis.

Possible Causes: Commonly occurs spontaneously, particularly in children. In dry environments or during winter months the membranes lining the nose may become dry and cracked causing a bleed. Injury to the nose can also cause bleeding. Other causes include forceful nose-blowing, the presence of a foreign body in the nose, infection of the upper respiratory tract, the use of anticoagulant drugs, hypertension, or an underlying medical condition such as cancer of the nasopharynx.

General Signs and Symptoms: Bleeding from the nose, usually from just one nostril.

Conventional Medical Treatment: Bleeds are usually minor and stop themselves. Putting direct pressure on both sides of the nose to squeeze the nostrils together and holding if for about 20 minutes whilst leaning forward and breathing through the mouth is often successful. Medical attention should be sought if heavy bleeding persists. The focus of the treatment will be on stopping the bleed and finding the cause. Various procedures are available including packing the nose and cauterizing (sealing) the vessel causing the bleed.

Prognosis: Not usually serious but persistent severe bleeds must be investigated.

Holistic Advice: Don't pick the nose or blow it too hard. Protect the nose when playing sport.

Onychomycosis

Definition: Fungal nail infection.

Possible Causes: Spread of fungal skin infections, such as athlete's foot, to the nail. Moist, sweaty feet provide an ideal environment for the growth of fungi. Fingernail infections are often caused by a yeast called candida that can cause infections of the skin around the nails. Damaged skin surrounding the nail is more likely to become infected so those with damaged skin or nails are at greater risk, as are those with a weakened immune system.

General Signs and Symptoms: Thickened, discoloured nail that can turn white, black, yellow or green. Pieces of the brittle nail may fall off or the whole nail can be lost. The underlying and surrounding tissues can become inflamed and painful. Men suffer from onychomycosis more that women and the incidence increases with age.

Conventional Medical Treatment: Mild cases may not need treatment. When treatment is required antifungal tablets and antifungal nail paints can be used.

Prognosis: Can be treated and usually cured but treatment can take several months. If left untreated the infection can spread to other nails.

Holistic Advice: Look after the nails. Do not bite the nails or surrounding tissues. Wash the feet regularly and dry them properly. Change socks or tights every day. Boost the immune system.

Onychoysis

Definition: The loosening or separation of a nail from the nail bed.

Possible Causes: Can be caused by damage to the nail and prolonged immersion of the hands in water. Also associated with several conditions including psoriasis, dermatitis, lichen planus of the nail (itchy rash of small, raised, flat-topped lesions that are shiny and pink/purple), certain thyroid problems, bacterial infections and fungal infections. Can be a side effect of some drugs.

General Signs and Symptoms: Opaque or whitened portion on the nail shows the area of separation. The nail may become thicker, pitted and cracked. Separation usually starts at the tip of the nail and works back. The tissues underneath the nail may become infected, making the nail appear green.

Conventional Medical Treatment: When symptomatic of another disease, treating the underlying cause should improve the onycholysis.

Prognosis: Nails grow continually throughout life and so will grow back unless the nail bed is damaged.

Holistic Advice: Take care of nails, keep them short and avoid contact with irritants. When possible, wear gloves to avoid getting the nails wet.

Osteoarthritis

Definition: Arthritis literally means inflammation of a joint. Osteoarthritis is an inflammatory disease of one or more joints in which the cartilage degenerates. There are many types of arthritis but osteoarthritis is the most common. Rheumatoid arthritis is more severe but less common. In rheumatoid arthritis the body's immune system attacks and destroys the joint(s). We'll focus on osteoarthritis, because it affects about 8.5 million people in the UK.

Possible Causes: Cause it not fully known but there may be a genetic predisposition to developing the disease. It is brought on by a reduced ability of the body to repair a joint(s). The cartilage becomes worn and uneven and the bones become thicker and broader, causing stiffness and pain in the affected joint(s). It may be caused by excessive joint usage, congenital bone deformity or simply excessive wear and tear. It can follow injury (e.g. fracture), and can be brought on by other inflammatory diseases. Obesity and repetitive movements may also be triggers.

General Signs and Symptoms: Localized inflammation due to the bones rubbing together. The joints (often the knees, hips and finger joints) may be painful, swollen, stiff (particularly after rest until they get going again) and deformed causing a lack of mobility. Joints may crack and creak, develop bony growths and may also become misaligned.

Conventional Medical Treatment: Variety of painkillers and anti-inflammatory drugs can be used to treat the symptoms. Some painkillers can be applied topically and others (typically corticosteroids) can be injected directly into the joint. In severe instances, and when possible, surgery can be used to restore the cartilage, replace joints (commonly the hip and knee) or to fuse the joints (to make the joint stronger and less painful). Physiotherapy can help joint mobility.

Prognosis: There is no cure for arthritis, but drugs can help reduce the symptoms. Controlling weight, ensuring good posture and avoiding stress and injury to the joints can help. Exercise can help maintain the range of joint movement and strengthen the muscles to better support the joints.

Holistic Advice: Avoid red meats, pork products, tea, coffee and alcohol. The supplements chondroitin and glucosamine are commonly taken. Take gentle exercise. Consider acupuncture and aromatherapy massage. Always treat the whole person. Look at the cause of any stress, any obesity and diet.

Osteogenesis Imperfecta

Definition: Genetic disorder characterised by bones that break easily. Also known as brittle bone disease.

Possible Causes: Caused by a genetic defect that affects the body's ability to make strong bones. This is usually because of a type I collagen deficiency. Type I collagen is normally the most abundant collagen in the body.

General Signs and Symptoms: Bones break easily for little or no obvious reason. Some may experience just a few fractures in a lifetime, others may experience hundreds. It may also cause weak muscles, brittle teeth, a curved spine and hearing loss. There are several types of osteogenesis imperfecta and they are used to categorise the symptoms and severity of the condition.

Conventional Medical Treatment: There is no cure. The treatment focuses on increasing bone mass and muscle strength to help prevent fractures and maintain mobility, as well as controlling the pain associated with fractures. Sufferers are encouraged to exercise as much as possible. Swimming is of particular value as the risk of fracture whilst participating in this form of exercise is small. Walking is also encouraged, even if mobility aids (such as braces and crutches) are required. A surgical procedure called "rodding" can be used, in which metal rods are inserted through the long bones to increase their strength and help prevent and/or correct any deformities.

Prognosis: Depends on the severity of each case.

Holistic Advice: Do everything possible to avoid depleting bone mass by not smoking, and not drinking excess caffeine and alcohol. Eat a balanced, healthy diet and lose any excess weight.

Osteomalacia

Definition: A disorder characterised by weak, soft bones that become distorted or facture easily. In children this condition is called rickets.

Possible Causes: The most common cause of osteomalacia is a deficiency of vitamin D or calcium – both vital for the formation of strong bones. Vitamin D is derived from exposure to sunlight and food such as oily fish, eggs and fortified cereals. Sources of calcium include dairy products, green vegetables and wholemeal bread. Children can also be born with a genetic form or rickets, and it can also be caused by underlying conditions that prevent the successful absorption of vitamins and minerals. Risk factors include having a darker skin type (which requires more sunlight for the body to produce sufficient quantities of vitamin D), being born prematurely, and taking medications that affect vitamin D.

General Signs and Symptoms: Rickets can cause bone pain, skeletal deformity, fragile bones that break easily, and dental problems, and it can inhibit growth and development. In adults, symptoms of osteomalacia include waddling when walking, bending bones, muscle weakness and muscle pain.

Conventional Medical Treatment: Rickets and osteomalacia caused by a lack of vitamin D and/or calcium in the diet is treated by dietary supplements, vitamin D injections, and dietary changes to increase the natural intake of vitamin D and calcium. If caused by an underlying medical condition, treating the condition will often help. In cases in which rickets has caused deformities such as bowed legs and curvature of the spine, surgery or the use of braces may be used to correct them, although some deformities may be permanent.

Prognosis: Taking supplements as directed will usually cure the condition although it may take several months before the bone pain and muscle weakness is relieved.

Holistic Advice: Osteomalacia and most cases of rickets can be avoided by ensuring the diet contains sufficient quantities of vitamin D and calcium. Most vitamin D comes from exposure to sunlight and just 15 minutes on the hands and face a few times a week in spring and summer is usually sufficient. Groups at risk of vitamin D deficiency (e.g. the elderly, housebound, those with dark skin and those who do not eat the vitamin D-rich foods) maybe advised to take supplements.

Osteoporosis

Definition: Reduced bone mass and increased porousness of the bone.

Possible Causes: As the body ages, more bone cells are lost than are replaced causing the bones to become thinner and weaker. Osteoporosis therefore develops slowly over several years. Women are at greater risk due to the decrease in oestrogen (essential for healthy bones) levels after the menopause. In men, testosterone helps to maintain healthy bones and so males with a lower level of this hormone may be more susceptible. Osteoporosis is also symptomatic of some diseases such as hyperthyroidism, disease of the renal glands, pituitary gland problems, arthritis, diabetes and renal failure. Lack of calcium salts, low levels of Vitamin D, poor nutrition, heavy drinking, smoking, some drugs and immobilization can also be risk factors. It can be familial.

General Signs and Symptoms: Increased risk of bone fractures. Often breaking a bone under circumstances which would not normally cause a fracture is the first sign of the condition, and tests carried out then result in the diagnosis. It can cause spinal crush, causing pain and loss of height.

Conventional Medical Treatment: Hormone replacement therapy may be recommended to increase the oestrogen level in woman, and men can be given testosterone treatment. Calcitonin can be given to inhibit the cells that break down bone. Other drugs can be used to help maintain bone density, and calcium and vitamin D supplements may be prescribed.

Prognosis: The body, particularly in the elderly, may not be able to heal the fractures effectively, so it can cause long term issues. As the bones weaken and give way, the condition itself may increase the likelihood of falls, so exacerbating the problem.

Holistic Advice: Seek nutritional advice regarding supplements and dairy intake. Maintain a healthy diet that contains calcium, stop smoking and limit alcohol intake. Regular exercise, including weight-bearing exercises, can help maintain bone strength and help prevent this condition.

Parkinson's Disease

Definition: A progressive brain disorder characterized by tremors, rigidity and impairment of voluntary movement.

Possible Causes: Parkinson's disease is characterised by low levels of the neurotransmitter dopamine. The reduction of the dopamine level is due to the loss of nerve cells in a part of the brain called the substantia nigra that are responsible for producing dopamine. The correct balance of dopamine and another neurotransmitter called acetylcholine is necessary for fine muscle control and smooth movement. It is not known why these brain cells are lost but it may be due to genetic and/or environmental factors.

General Signs and Symptoms: Slowness of movement, lack of co-ordination, difficulty with fine movements, tremors and muscle rigidity are the most typical symptoms. In the early signs the tremors tend to affect only one hand, arm or leg, usually at rest, and then later both sides are affected. The face may also lose its natural movement and the voice may alter due to the muscles of the larynx, tongue and lips changing. Speech may become impaired and there may be difficultly swallowing. Sufferers may also suffer from tiredness, depression and continence problems. The symptoms usually begin slowly and then gradually develop but in no particular order. Parkinson's affects everybody differently. It is more common in men than women, and is more likely after the age of 60.

Conventional Medical Treatment: Various drugs can be used to try to balance the levels of neurotransmitters in the brain to help relieve the symptoms. Anticholinergic drugs (given to help reduce muscular spasms) may also help reduce shaking and stiffness. Specialists may be needed to assist mobility, speech, continence and any psychological problems. Surgery is occasionally used on young suffers.

Prognosis: There is no cure. The treatments are available to help control the symptoms but cannot change the progression of the disease. Although many can lead an active life for many years after diagnosis, most will eventually need daily help and symptoms may get harder to treat.

Holistic Advice: Yoga can be beneficial to counteract the stiffening process. Promote a regular sleeping pattern, take regular exercise and maintain a healthy diet. Help groups can give valuable support and advice.

Paronychia

Definition: Infection of the fold of skin that surrounds a nail.

Possible Causes: Acute paronychia comes on quickly and is caused by a bacterial infection that enters the body through a cut or break in the skin that makes up the nail fold. Biting the nails can therefore make infection more likely. Those with decreased resistance to infection due to other underlying conditions are more susceptible. Chronic paronychia can develop over months and is common in those who have their hands in water for prolonged periods. The skin around the nail separates from the nail, softens, and then becomes infected usually by a yeast organism.

General Signs and Symptoms: Pain, swelling and redness in the infected area. The swelling may be filled with pus. Infection can spread to the fingertip causing finger pulp infection. If left untreated the nail may separate from the nail bed.

Conventional Medical Treatment: Antibiotics or antifungal drugs to treat the infection. Pus filled swellings may need to be drained.

Prognosis: Usually clears up quickly with treatment.

Holistic Advice: Anything to boost the immune system will help. Keep hands dry when possible, and maintain good hand hygiene.

Peptic Ulcers

Definition: An open sore on the lining of the stomach (gastric ulcer) or on the lining of the first part of the small intestine (duodenal ulcer).

Possible Causes: The majority of peptic ulcers are due to an infection by the Helicobacter pylori bacteria. These bacteria damage the protective mucus lining of the stomach and small intestine, leaving the underlying tissue subject to erosion by the acidic digestive juices, allowing an open sore to form. Peptic ulcers can also be caused by the long term use of some drugs such as aspirin and ibuprofen, which damage the stomach lining. Risk factors include family history, smoking, and alcohol consumption. Stress may worsen the symptoms.

General Signs and Symptoms: The most common symptom is burning pain or discomfort in the upper abdomen. There may also be loss of appetite, weight loss, a feeling of fullness in the abdomen, nausea and sometimes vomiting. The pain can be worse before meals when the stomach is empty.

Conventional Medical Treatment: Antibiotics can be used if the condition is caused by a bacterial infection. Antacids can help relieve the symptoms and a variety of drugs are available to help reduce the acidity, giving the ulcers time to heal. If the ulcers are caused by medication, a change of drugs will be considered. Tests may be carried out to rule out any more serious conditions.

Prognosis: The ulcer may bleed, causing a loss of blood, or perforate through the wall of the digestive tract allowing its contents into the abdomen. This can cause peritonitis (inflammation of the lining of the abdomen) and can be fatal. The inflammation may also cause gastric obstruction.

Holistic Advice: Make lifestyle changes to reduce stress. Cut down on alcohol and caffeine and stop smoking. Boost the immune system to help protect against infection.

Pernicious Anaemia

Definition: Anaemia is the term used to describe disorders in which the haemoglobin in the red blood cells is deficient or abnormal. Pernicious anaemia is an autoimmune disease that affects the stomach, preventing the absorption of vitamin B_{12}. Vitamin B_{12} is one of the necessary components required to produce healthy red blood cells.

Possible Causes: Vitamin B_{12} can only be absorbed from ingested food if it combines with a chemical called the intrinsic factor, which is produced by cells in the stomach. This autoimmune condition attacks the stomach cells, effectively stopping them from secreting the intrinsic factor. This leads to a deficiency in vitamin B_{12} and, as a result, the body produces abnormally large red blood cells that are unable to transport sufficient oxygen to the tissues. Risk factors include being female, being over 60, family history and having another autoimmune disorder. Pernicious anaemia is just one cause of vitamin B_{12} deficiency anaemia.

General Signs and Symptoms: General symptoms of anaemia include tiredness, lethargy, weakness, shortness of breath, palpitations, headache and faintness. Anaemia caused by vitamin B_{12} deficiency also has symptoms including jaundice, loss of balance, disturbed vision and an altered sense of touch. It can also have psychological effects.

Conventional Medical Treatment: Vitamin B_{12} levels can be boosted by regular injections. This will be a lifelong treatment.

Prognosis: Complications are rare but a long-term deficiency of vitamin B_{12} can cause problems.

Holistic Advice: Increasing the vitamin B_{12} in the diet has no effect, but eating a healthy, balanced diet can help ensure the sufficient supply of other vital vitamins.

Pertussis

Definition: Infection of the lining of the airways that causes bouts of coughing. Commonly called whooping cough.

Possible Causes: Caused by the Bordetella pertussis bacteria, which infect the trachea and the bronchi. The infection is highly infectious and transmitted in airborne droplets produced when infected people cough and sneeze.

General Signs and Symptoms: Typified by violent fits of coughing that end in a "whoop" when the person inhales. The symptoms may take up to 20 days to appear after infection. The symptoms resemble the common cold at first, and then worsen and the "whooping" cough develops. This may be accompanied by the production of large amounts of sputum. The severe coughing may cause vomiting and the rupture of small blood vessels, resulting in a rash of small, flat, red spots, especially around the face, hairline and eyes. The coughing can be very tiring, particularly for young children. Whooping cough usually affects infants and young children although adults can be affected.

Conventional Medical Treatment: The infection is treated with antibiotics. Seriously ill children may require hospitalisation. The pertussis vaccine is usually given routinely in childhood to protect from this condition.

Prognosis: Most make a full recovery but it can be life threatening in the very young.

Holistic Advice: The infection is highly infectious so great care must be taken not to spread the disease. Take plenty of rest and drink plenty of fluids.

Pharyngitis

Definition: Inflammation of the pharynx (throat), often described simply as a sore throat.

Possible Causes: Commonly caused by a viral infection, such as the common cold, or by a bacterial infection, such as the streptococcal bacteria. Smoking and alcohol may cause the throat to become sore, and a sore throat is sometimes symptomatic of another disease.

General Signs and Symptoms: The sore throat is usually accompanied by difficulty swallowing, swollen tonsils, enlarged neck glands, runny nose, headache, muscle aches and a cough.

Conventional Medical Treatment: Painkillers can help relieve the symptoms, as can throat lozenges containing local anaesthetic.

Prognosis: Pharyngitis usually clears up without treatment within 3-7 days. In severe cases it may cause breathing difficulties. It can develop into a more serious condition if the immune system is compromised.

Holistic Advice: Eating ice cream can help sooth the soreness. Drinking plenty of hot or very cold fluids can help. Hot lemon and honey drinks are good soothers. Using a humidifier to keep the surrounding air moist can be useful. Boost the immune system.

Pleurisy

Definition: Inflammation of the pleura.

Possible Causes: The two pleural membranes, which cover the lungs and separate the lungs from the chest wall, usually slide over each other to allow the lungs to inflate and deflate smoothly. Inflammation prevents this, and they rub together. The resulting friction causes sharp, severe chest pain when inhaling. Can be caused by a viral illness (e.g. flu), autoimmune disorders (e.g. rheumatoid arthritis) and injury to the ribs. Lung damage beneath the pleura, caused by conditions such as pneumonia, pulmonary embolism and lung cancer, can also cause the pleura to become inflamed.

General Signs and Symptoms: Sharp chest pain when inhaling deeply, coughing or sneezing (possibly restricted to just one side depending on the location of the pleurisy). There may be difficulty in breathing and a dry cough. The presence of a fever, a productive cough, serious breathing difficulties or a swollen arm or leg, may indicate a serious underlying condition for which medical attention should be sought quickly. When caused by infection or a pulmonary embolism, the symptoms can have a fast onset. In other cases the symptoms may occur gradually.

Conventional Medical Treatment: Non-steroidal anti-inflammatory drugs to relieve the pain and inflammation. Treatment will also be required for any underlying medical condition.

Prognosis: The condition generally clears up within 7-10 days of the start of treatment.

Holistic Advice: Holding the affected side during coughing may help ease the pain.

Pneumonia

Definition: Inflammation of the lung tissue in one or both lungs.

Possible Causes: The alveoli become inflamed and fill with fluid. This makes it difficult for oxygen to pass into the bloodstream. Inflammation is usually caused by bacterial infection, most commonly Streptococcus pneumoniae, but can be caused by other organisms including viruses and, more rarely, fungi. It can also be caused by breathing something into the lungs that causes an irritation, e.g. vomit, food, smoke or chemicals. There is an increased risk of developing this condition if the immune system is compromised, and those who are already seriously ill, malnourished, smoke or abuse alcohol are also more vulnerable. Legionnaires' disease is a form of pneumonia. It is caused by bacteria that are spread through air-conditioning systems.

General Signs and Symptoms: Pneumonia is typified by a cough that may be dry, but if productive produces thick yellow, green, brown or blood-stained mucus. There may be chest pain that is worse on inhalation, shortness of breath at rest, rapid heartbeat, fever, sweating, shivering and loss of appetite. The symptoms may have a fast or gradual onset depending on the cause.

Conventional Medical Treatment: If caused by a bacterial infection, antibiotics can be prescribed. Painkillers may help the pain and reduce any fever. For mild viral pneumonia no drug treatment is usually required. For severe infections, hospitalization may be necessary.

Prognosis: Although mild cases can usually be treated successfully at home, pneumonia can be fatal, particularly in infants and the elderly. Increasing resistance of some organisms to antibiotics is making some forms of pneumonia harder to treat.

Holistic Advice: Stop smoking. Drink plenty of fluids. Warm lemon and honey drinks may help ease the discomfort caused by coughing. Higher risk groups can be vaccinated against this condition.

Poliomyelitis

Definition: Highly infectious disease that can attack the nerves which may lead to muscle paralysis. Poliomyelitis has been eradicated in the UK but remains a serious problem in India, Pakistan, Afghanistan and Nigeria. It is often simply referred to as polio.

Possible Causes: Caused by a virus called enterovirus. It thrives in the gastrointestinal tract and then may move to the nervous system. It is spread by oral contact with faeces from an infected person, commonly through contaminated water and food.

General Signs and Symptoms: For most it is asymptomatic, or only results in a mild illness with a slight fever, sore throat, nausea, vomiting, diarrhoea and constipation. In less than 1%, paralysis may result. The first symptoms of the paralytic form include fever, headache, back and neck stiffness, constipation and increased sensitivity to touch. The damage to the nerve cells leads to muscle weakness, and the limbs may become loose and floppy. Difficulties may be experienced with the senses (sight, sound, smell, taste and touch) and the heart muscle and respiratory muscles may also be affected.

Conventional Medical Treatment: There is no cure and so vaccination is very important to prevent the disease. The treatment can only help to ease the symptoms experienced. Mild cases may be treated with rest and painkillers. Physiotherapy may help speed recovery if the muscles have been affected. Severe cases may require a ventilator to assist breathing.

Prognosis: Most make a full recovery from mild forms of the disease. Many of those who become paralysed improve within 6 months, but some can be left with permanent paralysis and deformity. It has been found that a large percentage of those who contracted polio suffer from post-polio syndrome many years after the infection. Symptoms of post-polio syndrome include fatigue, muscle weakness and muscle and joint pain.

Holistic Advice: Ensure vaccines are up to date before travelling to parts of the world where poliomyelitis is still a risk. A booster may be required.

Polycystic Ovary Syndrome

Definition: Multiple, small, fluid-filled cysts in the ovaries.

Possible Causes: The cause in unknown but it is associated with resistance to insulin and sex hormone imbalance. Resistance to insulin causes more to be produced. This increased level of insulin causes the ovaries to produce too much testosterone which interferes with the development of the follicle, prevents normal ovulation and may create "masculine" symptoms such as the increased growth of body hair. It also causes weight gain. Many women with this condition have raised levels in luteinising hormone, follicle stimulating hormone and prolactin, and lower levels of thyroid hormones. This condition tends to run in families and there are connections to a family history of diabetes and high cholesterol. Obesity is a major risk factor.

General Signs and Symptoms: The condition may cause irregular ovulation or prevent it altogether. Sufferers may experience irregular or light periods and infertility problems. Other possible symptoms include the excessive growth of body hair, acne, depression and weight gain. Symptoms may vary in severity and the condition may go unnoticed until tests are carried out to explain the cause of infertility.

Conventional Medical Treatment: The treatment depends on the severity of the symptoms and if the woman wants to conceive. Lifestyles changes can significantly help, particularly losing excess weight. Hormone treatment can be given to reduce testosterone levels which helps to regulate periods and reduce the "maleness" symptoms. Creams can also be used to slow down hair growth. Diabetes drugs can help to treat the insulin resistance and increase ovulation. Fertility drugs can promote fertility. A surgical procedure can use heat or laser on the ovaries to destroy the tissue that is creating the male hormones. Topical treatments can be used to help relieve the symptom of acne.

Prognosis: Cannot be cured but the symptoms can be treated and fertility improved. Left untreated it can lead to type 2 diabetes mellitus, hypertension and high cholesterol levels. There is a greater risk of endometrial cancer in those who have not regularly menstruated for many years.

Holistic Advice: Lose excess weight and exercise regularly. Ensure a healthy balanced diet.

Postnatal Depression

Definition: Depressive feelings or psychological disturbances in the first few weeks or months after childbirth.

Possible Causes: Depression is often triggered by emotional and stressful events. Childbirth tends to be both of these. Postnatal depression was thought to be caused by a fall in hormone levels but now it is thought likely to be caused by a combination of environmental, psychological, physical and emotional factors. Risk factors include previous experiences of depression, family history, feelings of inadequacy and isolation, concerns about new responsibilities, lack of support, relationship or financial worries, lack of sleep, stress, a difficult labour, and physical problems post-birth.

General Signs and Symptoms: The usual symptoms of depression are commonly present, e.g. low self esteem, tearfulness and feelings of despair. The sufferer may feel unable to cope, have panic attacks and dramatic mood swings, experience a lack of motivation and lack of interest in anything (including the baby), and be tired and irritable. Some women also get thoughts about harming their baby.

Conventional Medical Treatment: The earlier the condition is recognized the better. Just admitting to the feelings and talking about them can help. Antidepressants may be prescribed and counselling may be recommended. In very severe cases, where it is thought the baby or mother may be at risk from harm, hospitalisation or admission to a mental health clinic may be required. Electroconvulsive therapy may be recommended if all other treatments have failed.

Prognosis: As long as it is recognised and treated, it is a short-term condition from which a full recovery can be made.

Holistic Advice: Get as much rest and relaxation as possible, take gentle, regular exercise, eat regular, healthy meals, avoid alcohol and talk about feelings. Local support groups can offer help.

Premenstrual Syndrome

Definition: Various symptoms that may affect women in the days leading up to menstruation.

Possible Causes: The exact cause is unknown, but it is thought to be due to hormonal and chemical changes associated with menstruation. A chemical called serotonin, known to regulate mood, fluctuates during the menstrual cycle. Low levels may contribute to tiredness, food cravings and insomnia. Risk factors may include being overweight, stress, caffeine, alcohol and chocolate.

General Signs and Symptoms: Vary between women and may change month to month. Symptoms can be physical (e.g. fluid retention, bloating, breast tenderness, abdominal pain, tiredness, headaches or migraine, backache and muscle stiffness), psychological (e.g. mood swings, feeling irritable, depression and difficulty concentrating) and behavioural (e.g. loss of interest in sex and changes in appetite).

Conventional Medical Treatment: Self help measures are encouraged to ensure diet and the level of exercise taken are optimized to reduce risk factors. Failing that, medications such as non-steroidal anti-inflammatories (to ease sore breasts, headaches and muscular pain), diuretic drugs (to reduce water retention and bloating), oral contraceptives and synthetic hormones (to help regulate hormonal activity) and some antidepressant drugs (to help with the psychological effects) can be prescribed. If many symptoms are psychological, therapies such as cognitive behavioural therapy may also be of use.

Prognosis: There is no cure but treatments help the symptoms to be managed.

Holistic Advice: Any therapy that can help reduce stress and promote relaxation may be of benefit. Some find supplements of evening primrose oil and vitamin B6 (very high doses can be harmful) may help. Chamomile tea is calming and diuretic which can help relieve the water retention. Maintain a good, balanced, high fibre, fresh food diet, cutting down on saturated fats, sugar, salt and caffeine. Take regular exercise and try to stay stress free.

Prolapsed Intervertebral Disc

Definition: Protrusion of one of the shock-absorbing pads that lie between the vertebrae. Also known as a slipped disc.

Possible Causes: Intervertebral discs have a strong fibrous outer layer and a soft, gelatinous inner. A prolapsed disc occurs when the gel inside the core pushes outwards, distorting the shape of the disc. The outer coat can rupture, allowing the gel to leak out. The damaged disc can put pressure on an individual nerve or the whole spinal cord creating pain in any part of the body served by the affected nerve. Risk factors that may decrease the strength of the supporting connective tissue that holds the disc in place include age, awkward bending, heavy lifting, sitting for long periods, smoking, being overweight and having a back injury. Once weakened, the disc may slip.

General Signs and Symptoms: Most will experience pain, often beginning in the back and radiating to other parts of the body depending on which nerve is under pressure from the prolapsed disc. It can cause muscular weakness and spasm. The sciatic nerve is commonly affected, leading to sciatic pain that runs from the back of the pelvis, through the buttocks and down one or both legs, causing aching, numbness and tingling.

Conventional Medical Treatment: Given time the disc will often shrink back and so the pain ceases. Medication such as painkillers, non-steroidal anti-inflammatory drugs, corticosteroid injections and muscle relaxants may be prescribed to cope with the pain. In severe cases surgery may be recommended to remove the pressure on the nerve caused by the slipped disc.

Prognosis: For most, a combination of gentle exercise and painkillers will resolve the situation within about 4-6 weeks but it can be a serious problem and once there is a weakness, the condition may recur.

Holistic Advice: Regular exercise to keep the back strong and flexible, and ensuring that correct lifting techniques are used can help prevent this condition. Maintaining a good posture at all times, sleeping on a suitable mattress and not carrying any excess body weight also contribute to keeping the spine healthy and functional.

Prostatitis

Definition: Inflammation of the prostate gland. There are 3 main types – acute prostatitis, chronic bacterial prostatitis and chronic non-bacterial prostatitis.

Possible Causes: Acute prostatitis is uncommon and is caused by bacteria that enter the prostate from the urinary tract. Chronic prostatitis is also caused by bacterial infection of the prostate, but in this case the bacteria infection develops in the prostate and may then spread into the urinary tract. Chronic non bacterial prostatitis is the most common. Its cause is unknown but may be linked to problems in the immune system or nervous system, or from an undiscovered viral or bacterial infection.

General Signs and Symptoms: Acute prostatitis produces sudden and severe symptoms including a fever and severe pain in the pelvis, genitals, lower back, base of the penis and the buttocks. There may be a need to urinate frequently and urination, ejaculation and defaecation may be painful. Chronic prostatitis does not always show symptoms, but if symptoms do occur they tend to develop gradually and be mild but persistent, although they can fluctuate in severity from day to day. The symptoms for chronic prostatitis are the same as for acute prostatitis but some may also experience tiredness, joint and muscle pain.

Conventional Medical Treatment: Antibiotics can be used to treat cases of prostatitis caused by bacterial infection. Alpha blockers may also be used to relax the bladder muscles to help with urination. Laxatives can be used to help bowel movement. Non-bacterial prostatitis can be difficult to treat because of the lack of knowledge about its cause. Alpha blockers, paracetamol and ibuprofen are commonly prescribed to help treat the symptoms.

Prognosis: Most men make a full recovery but all types of prostatitis can recur.

Holistic Advice: Any prostate problem should be checked out to eliminate any sinister underlying cause.

Psoriasis

Definition: Inflammatory skin disorder.

Possible Causes: It is believed that the immune system may play a part by attacking healthy skin cells by mistake. There is an increased production of epidermal cells that results in immature cells reaching the surface of the skin. Psoriasis is often a family disease. It can be triggered by immune-depressing influences such as stress. Other triggers can include injury to skin, alcohol, smoking, some medicines and some immune disorders. Can be seasonal, in which case it is especially prevalent in spring and autumn.

General Signs and Symptoms: Raised, flaky, reddened, crusty areas covered with silvery scales, and chronic inflammation. Often appears on elbows, knees and scalp. The disease is divided into several varieties according to the shape and distribution of the patches.

Conventional Medical Treatment: Topical creams and ointments, phototherapy (exposing skin to certain types of ultraviolet light), oral and injected medication that reduces the production of skin cells.

Prognosis: Long-lasting (chronic) disease that can return at any time. There is no cure but the range of treatments can help alleviate symptoms. It is often cyclical, causing problems for a few weeks or month and then easing or stopping.

Holistic Advice: Stress must be treated. Anything that can help boost the immune system may help. Emollient creams can help to reduce scaliness. Eating raw vegetables and fresh fruit and drinking plenty of water can also be beneficial.

Pulmonary Embolism

Definition: Obstruction of the blood flow to the lungs by one or more blood clots.

Possible Causes: A plug of material, called an embolus, gets lodged in a pulmonary artery, either partially or completely blocking the flow of blood. The word embolism refers to the blockage of an artery by the embolus. The embolus is usually made from pieces of a blood clot that have separated from a larger clot (thrombis) somewhere else in the body (often the legs) and travelled to the lungs in the bloodstream. Blood clots can be caused by slow blood flow, blood that clots too easily and blood vessel damage. Those with deep vein thrombosis (DVT) are at greater risk of pulmonary embolism. Other risk factors include inactivity, age, previous clots, family history, cancer and its treatments, combined contraceptive pill, hormone replacement therapy, pregnancy and obesity.

General Signs and Symptoms: Symptoms depend on the extent of the blockage. A large clot that prevents the flow of blood can cause sudden death. Single, very small clots may be asymptomatic. In most cases symptoms include shortness of breath, sharp chest pain, feeling faint and palpitations. The symptoms develop suddenly over a few minutes.

Conventional Medical Treatment: Treatment depends on the extent of the blockage. Anticoagulant drugs, such as heparin and warfarin, are usually given to help prevent existing clots from getting bigger and new clots from forming. Long term use of anticoagulants may be required. Emergency surgery may even be needed to remove the clot.

Prognosis: 1 in 3 massive pulmonary embolisms result in death. Those that survive the first few days are likely to make a full recovery. Those with recurrent minor pulmonary embolism may remain short of breath.

Holistic Advice: This is a medical emergency requiring urgent hospitalisation. The risk can be reduced by not smoking, losing any excess weight, taking regular exercise and eating a balanced healthy diet.

Pyelonephritis

Definition: Kidney infection resulting in the inflammation of one or both of the kidneys. Because the kidneys are a part of the urinary tract, pyelonephritis is classed as a urinary tract infection (UTI).

Possible Causes: Usually caused by a bacterial infection (typically e-coli bacteria that live in the colon) that gets transferred from the anus to the urethra and then moves up from the bladder to the kidney(s). Occasionally a kidney infection can develop from a bacterial or fungal skin infection, and bacteria may also be carried to the kidneys in the blood. Other risk factors include blockages of the urinary tract, kidney stones, conditions that prevent the bladder from fully emptying and a weakened immune system. People with diabetes mellitus are more likely to suffer from urinary tract infections because the presence of glucose in the urine may encourage bacterial growth. Pyelonephritis can also be caused if bacteria are introduced to the urinary tract during catheterization. Women, particularly those who are sexually active, are at greater risk.

General Signs and Symptoms: Typical symptoms include a fever, shivering, pain in the side of the abdomen, nausea, vomiting, diarrhoea and back pain. Symptoms usually develop quickly. If other parts of the urinary tract are affected symptoms associated with cystitis can also be experienced, e.g. cloudy or strong smelling urine, a feeling of incomplete emptying of the bladder, blood in the urine, and lower abdominal pain.

Conventional Medical Treatment: Antibiotics are used to tackle the infection. Any underlying cause may also be treated.

Prognosis: Most recover fully within about 2 weeks.

Holistic Advice: Drink plenty of fluids. Empty the bladder frequently and completely. After going to the toilet wipe from front to back, wash before and after sex, and urinate after sex.

Raynaud's

Definition: Sudden, intermittent narrowing of the arteries in the hands or, rarely, the feet.

Possible Causes: Muscular spasm of the artery walls restricts the blood supply to the fingers or toes. In most cases it is not caused by an underlying condition and is therefore called primary Raynaud's. Secondary Raynaud's is caused by an underlying condition, particularly scleroderma (thickening of the skin) and autoimmune conditions such as rheumatoid arthritis and lupus. Risk factors include exposure to the cold, side effect of some medications, exposure to vibration, smoking, stress, anxiety and injury or overuse of the fingers.

General Signs and Symptoms: Fingers or toes become pale and then blue and feel numb or tingly. The fingers or toes become very red as the blood returns to the tissues. It may cause a painful burning sensation. In primary Raynaud's all the fingers on both hands are usually affected at once. In secondary Raynaud's symptoms often begin only on a couple of fingers on one hand. Raynaud's is most common in women aged 15-45 and is usually mild.

Conventional Medical Treatment: Preventative measures such as keeping warm and not smoking may be sufficient to deal with mild symptoms. In severe cases medication can be given to dilate the small blood vessels, and a surgical procedure can be used to cut or strip out the nerves to the affected area to reduce the pain. As a last resort, intravenous infusion therapy can be used to introduce a drug into the body that dilates the small blood vessels and helps prevent blood clotting. For secondary Raynaud's, the underlying cause of the problem will be investigated and, if found, it will be treated accordingly.

Prognosis: Usually harmless but severe cases may lead to skin ulcers or gangrene on the tips of the digits affected.

Holistic Advice: Keep warm, avoid direct contact with cold objects, reduce caffeine intake and give up smoking.

Rheumatoid Arthritis

Definition: Chronic autoimmune disease that causes the joints to become painful, swollen, stiff and deformed.

Possible Causes: The immune system attacks the lining of the joints, causing swelling and inflammation. If the inflammation persists it may damage the ends of the bone and the cartilage that covers them. Tendons and ligaments may also become worn and deformity of the joint arises. The actual cause of this autoimmune condition is unknown. Some think it may be triggered by an infection or virus but nothing is proven. It is more common in women and so oestrogen may play a part. There is some evidence that it may run in families.

General Signs and Symptoms: The condition causes joint pain, stiffness and warmth and redness in the affected area. The joints may appear bumpy. Rheumatoid arthritis tends to develop slowly with the small joints, commonly in the hands, being affected first. The condition has "flare-ups" and the symptoms tend to worsen with each one. The pain and stiffness is usually worse in the mornings. Other general symptoms such as tiredness, poor appetite and loss of weight may show and, because the condition can be painful and debilitating, depression is quite common.

Conventional Medical Treatment: There is no cure. The treatment focuses on controlling the symptoms and reducing further joint damage by slowing the progression of the disease. Many different drugs are available, some for the pain and some to slow the progression of the disease. Surgery can be used to correct joint deformities and reduce pain. Physiotherapy and, as the disease progresses, help with day-to-day life may be necessary.

Prognosis: Lifelong drug treatment may be needed to control the symptoms. Some will become severely disabled. Complications include carpal tunnel syndrome, ruptured tendons and bursitis, and the inflammation may affect other parts of the body including the lungs, heart, blood vessels and the eyes.

Holistic Advice: Take gentle, regular exercise and maintain a healthy diet. Support groups can offer advice and self-help guidance for the sufferer and his/her family.

<u>Scars</u>

Definition: A patch or line of tissue that remains after a wound has healed. Can be internal and external.

Possible Causes: Natural part of healing process that occurs after body tissue has been damaged, in which the body produces more of the protein collagen. Abnormal scars can develop if the wound becomes infected, when there is a loss of a large patch of skin, and after serious burns.

General Signs and Symptoms: External scars are visible. Scarring can be worse on more mobile areas of the body that continue to move during the healing process. Scars gradually become smoother and softer. Abnormal scars can be itchy, painful and unsightly.

Conventional Medical Treatment: Drugs may be prescribed to help break down scar tissue. Laser treatment and surgery can be used on severe cases to improve the appearance.

Prognosis: The affect a scar has on the person's life is largely dependent on how they feel about it. Scars tend to fade with time but can have detrimental psychological effects.

Holistic Advice: Creams or supplements containing vitamin E can speed up the healing process. Eggs and leafy green vegetables are rich in vitamin E. Make-up can be used to camouflage scars. How the person feels about themselves and the impact the scar has on their life should be addressed. The severity of the scarring can be minimized at the time of the injury by keeping the wound clean. Don't pick scabs or spots!

Sciatica

Definition: Pain originating from the sciatic nerve.

Possible Causes: Sciatica results from the compression or damage to the sciatic nerve or its roots. This can be brought on by a slipped disc, narrowing of the spinal cord, degeneration of the intervertebral discs, osteoarthritis, muscle spasm, injury and additional pressure on the spine during pregnancy, but sometimes the cause is unknown.

General Signs and Symptoms: Pain in the lower back and buttock that travels down the back of the thigh and outside of the leg, often going into the outside of the foot. May cause numbness, muscle weakness or tingling in the legs and feet. Movement usually makes the pain worse.

Conventional Medical Treatment: Acute (short-term) sciatica can usually be managed with a combination of painkillers, anti-inflammatory drugs, exercise and hot/cold packs. In more severe cases stronger painkillers may be necessary and physiotherapy or chiropractic may be required. Surgery can be used to reduce the pressure on the sciatic nerve by removing discs, fusing vertebrae, or by widening the spinal cord.

Prognosis: Mild sciatica does not usually last longer than 6 weeks and tends to sort itself out without treatment. Sciatica can recur unless the underlying cause is rectified.

Holistic Advice: Look into general posture and the work/home environment e.g. height of chairs, desks and computer screen. The shortening of the piriformis muscle can often cause sciatic pain, so soft tissue manipulation (including muscle energy techniques) can also be beneficial. Bed rest may provide temporary relief but can make the symptoms worse. Walking and gentle stretching is of benefit. Acupuncture may help relieve the pain. Some find regular "maintenance" visits to an osteopath or chiropractor beneficial.

Seasonal Affective Disorder

Definition: A type of depression that has a seasonal pattern. Often abbreviated to SAD.

Possible Causes: Thought to be linked to the reduced exposure to sunlight in the winter months. The lack of light may affect the hormones melatonin (influencing sleep patterns) and serotonin (affecting mood, appetite and sleep). Reduced sunlight may also affect the body's natural internal clock. Risk factors include family history of depression, adverse childhood experiences, and psychological and social factors.

General Signs and Symptoms: Depression is more apparent in the winter months, resulting in being less active, putting on weight and sleeping more. Sufferers may feel tired, stressed, anxious and generally unhappy. The usual symptoms of depression are commonly present, e.g. low self esteem, tearfulness and feelings of despair.

Conventional Medical Treatment: Antidepressants and the usual psychosocial treatments used for other forms of depression may help. Light therapy, to expose the body to more light during the winter months, may give short-term relief. This involves wearing a light visor or sitting in front of a light box.

Prognosis: Like any form of depression, it can be difficult to live with. Treatments can offer relief.

Holistic Advice: Try to get as much natural sunlight as possible, and make living and working environments light and bright. Take regular exercise, preferably outdoors, and eat a healthy, well balanced diet. Avoid stressful situations and talk to family and friends about feelings and concerns.

Sebaceous Cysts

Definition: A sebaceous cyst is a harmless swelling under the skin that may become infected. The term "cyst" is a general term used to describe an enclosed sac that may contain air, fluids or semi-solid material, but not normally pus. Cysts can appear in various locations of the body, e.g. ovarian cysts, epididymal cysts and breast cysts. Cysts are usually harmless but depending on their location can be malignant. We will focus on sebaceous cysts here.

Possible Causes: Commonly caused by the inflammation of a hair follicle (also called follicular cyst). The sac of the cyst fills with a fatty, white, semi-solid material made up of dead skin cells and sebum.

General Signs and Symptoms: A smooth, usually painless lump under the skin. Some cysts have a dark central pore. They commonly occur on the scalp, face, trunk and genitals but may appear anywhere. They may grow large and become unsightly. If a cyst gets infected by bacteria it can become inflamed and painful and may eventually burst.

Conventional Medical Treatment: Can be left untreated if the cyst is not causing problems. Should a cyst become infected, it can be treated with antibiotics or can be incised and drained. Problematic cysts can be surgically removed under local anaesthetic. If not completely removed they may return.

Prognosis: No serious health implications.

Holistic Advice: Boost the immune system. Maintain good skin hygiene.

Shingles

Definition: An infection of a nerve and the area of skin that follows its path.

Possible Causes: Caused by the herpes varicella-zoster virus. This virus also causes chickenpox and can remain dormant in nerve cells until triggered later in life. It is thought that stress or ill health may cause the reactivation of the virus. It most commonly occurs in those aged 50-70, and those with a reduced immunity are at greatest risk. The herpes varicella-zoster virus is contagious and, although it will not cause shingles in another, direct contact with open blisters, which typify shingles, may cause chicken pox in a person who is not immune to this disease.

General Signs and Symptoms: The early symptoms of tingling and localised pain are followed by a painful rash of blisters that erupt along a path of a nerve, typically only on one side of the body. It usually affects the skin on the chest, abdomen or face. Other symptoms may include a fever, myalgia and tiredness. The blisters form scabs within 3-4 days and drop off several days later, possibly leaving scars. Discomfort may continue long after the rash has disappeared. This pain is called postherpetic neuralgia.

Conventional Medical Treatment: Antiviral drugs may be prescribed and painkillers may be used to reduce the discomfort. Calamine lotion may help the rash, as may wearing loose fitting clothing and keeping the rash as clean as possible to avoid bacterial infection. Antihistamines may help to relieve the itching. Anticonvulsant drugs may be prescribed to ease any postherpetic neuralgia.

Prognosis: There is no cure but most recover within 4-6 weeks, although postherpetic neuralgia may last several months. The treatments can only help ease the symptoms. The infection may recur.

Holistic Advice: Try to maintain healthy immune system and reduce stress levels. Try to prevent spreading the virus by not sharing towels, playing contact sports or swimming.

Sinusitis

Definition: Inflammation of the lining of the sinuses.

Possible Causes: Commonly caused by a viral infection (e.g. common cold or flu) but can be bacterial. The resulting inflammation causes the sinuses to block which results in mucus collecting in them, which may then create a secondary bacterial infection. Sinusitis can also be triggered or worsened by irritants (e.g. smoke and air pollution), allergic conditions (e.g. hay fever and asthma) and anything that narrows the nasal passages (e.g. nasal polyps and structural defects). Sufferers of cystic fibrosis (which causes a build up of mucus in the body) are more likely to develop sinusitis. Those with reduced immunity are more susceptible to the infections that cause sinusitis.

General Signs and Symptoms: Facial pain, chronic dull ache around the cheekbones, blocked or runny nose, discoloured nasal discharge, headache (especially when the head tips forward), and a raised temperature. The sufferer may also feel tired and unwell and may experience a loss of taste and smell and develop a cough and bad breath.

Conventional Medical Treatment: Painkillers and decongestants can be used to relieve the facial pain and help the blocked nose. If symptoms persist, antibiotics may be given if there is a bacterial infection and steroid sprays or drops can help reduce the inflammation. Surgery can be performed to widen and improve the function of the sinuses.

Prognosis: Often clears up by itself within about two and a half weeks.

Holistic Advice: Avoid dairy and wheat products as they may provoke excessive formation of mucus. Consider regular massage to boost the immune system. Facial massage, concentrating on the sinus points, can help to clear the congestion. Acupuncture may be beneficial. Steam inhalation may help to release the mucus. Drink plenty of water, exercise regularly and do not smoke.

Snoring

Definition: Noisy breathing during sleep.

Possible Causes: The noise associated with snoring is created when the soft tissues at the back of the nose, mouth and throat vibrate as the person breathes. This may be caused by an obstruction or narrowing of the pharynx leading from the back of the nasal cavity to the throat. This may be worsened by being overweight and more likely if lying on the back. Another possible cause is the relaxation or swelling of the tissue of the soft palette. Relaxation can be caused by alcohol or sedatives, and swelling can be caused by a throat infection or irritation of the palette by tobacco smoke. The vibration caused by the snoring itself further narrows the airway. The narrowing of the airways is called upper airway resistance syndrome (UARS). Severe snoring may be related to obstructive sleep apnea (OSA), where the airways may block for several seconds. The oxygen level falls, causing the person to come out of the deep sleep in order for normal breathing to resume.

General Signs and Symptoms: Snoring is characterised by snorting or rattling noises when asleep. In mild cases the snoring does no harm but in some cases breathing difficulties are experienced. UARS and OSA may have a detrimental affect on health, causing heart disease and strokes. Snoring can interrupt sleep patterns, causing tiredness, reducing concentration levels and increasing the risk of accidents.

Conventional Medical Treatment: Treatment is only usually required if snoring is affecting day to day life. Lifestyle changes such as reducing alcohol intake, losing weight and not smoking is usually the first requirement. If lifestyles changes do not help, devices are available to fit inside the mouth or nose to help keep the airways open. There are several surgical techniques that can be used as a last resort.

Prognosis: It may be possible to reduce snoring but a complete cure may not be possible.

Holistic Advice: Make the lifestyles changes as indicated above. Try not to roll over onto the back – sewing a golf ball to the back of nightwear can help this! Don't ignore emotional wellbeing.

Spinal Disorders

General Information: The spine protects the spinal cord and normally forms a straight, vertical line when viewed from the back. When viewed from the side, it has 2 main curves. It curves outwards at the top of the spine and inwards in the lower back. Abnormal curvatures of the spine can limit mobility and severely affect posture which, in turn, puts additional strain on other parts of the body. People with abnormal curvatures have a predisposition to other spinal problems later in life such as prolapsed discs. Posture can often be improved by physiotherapy, which strengthens the muscles supporting the spine. Three common spinal disorders are summarised below:

Kyphosis: Excessive outward curvature at the top of the spine. This results in a rounded back or "hunchback". The cause is not known in childhood but, in adults, disorders that limit mobility, such as osteoarthritis, or those that weaken the vertebrae, such as osteoporosis, are the most common causes. It may also be caused by poor posture.

Lordosis: Excessive inward curvature in the lower back. This shows as a hollow back. Lordosis may develop in those with weak abdominal muscles and poor posture. Those who are overweight are at risk of lordosis because they tend to lean back to improve balance. Kyphosis can lead to lordosis, because the lower spine compensates for the imbalance caused by the curve at the top. Kyphosis and lordosis commonly occur together, resulting in an excessive curvature at both the top of the back and in the lower back.

Scoliosis: Abnormal sideways curvature of the spine. It most commonly affects the spine in the chest area and lower back. It is more common in females and if left untreated the deformity can worsen. The cause is often unknown but it can be familial and in some cases the scoliosis is congenital. It can be due to skeletal defects such as unequal leg length or, rarely, muscle weakness around the spine or a neuromuscular disease. If there is no underlying cause and the scoliosis is slight, the condition will be monitored. In severe cases a spinal brace may be required to limit further curvature and surgery may be required to fuse the affected vertebrae or to straighten the spine with metal rods and wires.

Sprains and Strains

Definition: A sprain is a stretched, twisted or torn ligament. A strain is a stretch or tear of a muscle.

Possible Causes: Injury, commonly sustained playing sport, in which the ligament or muscle is over-stretched and damaged.

General Signs and Symptoms: Sprains cause inflammation, pain and bruising around a joint. It may not be possible to put weight on the joint and its movement may be limited. The bruising may not appear immediately and when it does may be some distance from the injured joint. Strains cause pain, swelling and bruising in the affected muscle.

Conventional Medical Treatment: Usually treated from home, following the PRICE guidelines – protection, rest, ice, compression and elevation. In the case of sprains, it is considered of benefit to gently move the joint when the inflammation allows. With muscle strains, the muscle should be kept as still as possible for the first few days. Painkillers can be used to treat the pain.

Prognosis: Most sprains and strains will heal successfully. If the symptoms do not improve after a few days, medical attention should be sought.

Holistic Advice: Sprains and strains can be avoided to some extent by stretching and strengthening exercises. Warm up properly before exercise and strap weak joints.

Stroke

Definition: Damage to a part of the brain caused by an interruption in its blood supply.

Possible Causes: There are 2 main causes of a stroke. The most common is when a blood clot prevents blood from reaching the brain. This is called an ischaemic stroke. Risk factors include smoking, hypertension, obesity, high cholesterol level, diabetes, irregular heartbeat, family history of heart disease or diabetes, and drinking alcohol to excess. The term "transient ischaemic attack" (TIA) is given to a temporary interruption to the blood supply to the brain. These are often a warning signs that a full blown ischemic stroke is imminent. The other main type of stoke is a haemorrhagic stroke. In this case the stroke is caused by a blood vessel in the brain bursting. Risk factors include being overweight, lack of exercise, smoking, drinking too much alcohol, taking anticoagulant medication and head injury.

General Signs and Symptoms: Signs and symptoms vary from person to person but the crucial signs can be remembered by the acronym FAST:-
F – Face: may drop on one side, person unable to smile
A – Arms: may be unable to raise (or hold up for long) one or both arms
S – Speech: may be slurred or garbled
T - Time: to dial 999 – a stroke should be considered a medical emergency
There may also be numbness on one side of the body, clumsiness, visual disturbances, headache and vomiting.

Conventional Medical Treatment: The sooner a stroke can be diagnosed and the treatment started the greater the chance of a full recovery. For ischaemic strokes, medication is given to try to dissolve the clot. Anticoagulants may be used to help prevent further clots forming. Medications can be used to help reduce the risk factors by reducing blood pressure and bringing down cholesterol levels. Emergency surgery is often required for haemorrhagic strokes to remove the leaked blood and repair the damaged vessel. Physiotherapy may be required if the stroke has caused mobility problems. Some stroke victims are left with permanent disability and may require long-term nursing care.

Prognosis: Strokes are largely avoidable by making life changes. Most stroke victims make a full recovery but about a third is left with long term disability.

Holistic Advice: Eat a healthy, low fat diet, take regular exercise, reduce stress, give up smoking and do not drink alcohol to excess.

Superficial Thrombophlebitis

Definition: Inflammation of a vein, commonly a varicose vein, just below the surface of the skin that causes a blood clot. (Note: thrombus = blood clot, phlebitis = inflammation of a vein)

Possible Causes: Venous inflammation and the subsequent blood clot can be caused by damage to the vein, the slow flow of the blood, or blood that clots more readily than it should. Risk factors include varicose veins, long periods of inactivity, oral contraceptive pill, pregnancy, diabetes, liver disease, immunosuppressant medicines, surgery, intravenous drug injections, history of thrombosis, and cancer. This condition is more common in adult women and there could be a familial link.

General Signs and Symptoms: The skin overlying a vein may appear red, or a superficial vein may feel painful, tender, swollen and feel hard. A mild fever may be experienced. Although it can be painful, this condition is less serious than deep vein thrombosis. However, if the symptoms significantly worsen, and swelling or heat spreads up the leg, medical attention should be sought urgently.

Conventional Medical Treatment: Most cases improve in a few days without treatment. Painkillers may be used to treat the pain and the leg may feel more comfortable rested and raised. Compression stockings can help. If the condition is caused by the blood clotting too readily, anticoagulants may be prescribed. If a varicose vein causes repeated problems it may be removed.

Prognosis: Rarely it may spread up to a deep vein, leading to deep vein thrombosis.

Holistic Advice: Take regular gentle exercise, do not smoke and try to avoid getting varicose veins.

Tendonitis

Definition: Inflammation of a tendon.

Possible Causes: Overuse of a tendon or injury, often in the shoulder, elbow (tennis elbow), wrist, fingers, thigh, knee, or back of heel. It is more common in sportsmen, due to the risk of overuse and injury, and in the elderly because tendons become less elastic with age. Tendonitis is also more common in people with diabetes.

General Signs and Symptoms: Pain, a grating or cracking sensation, swelling, and weakness in the affected area. A lump may develop along the tendon.

Conventional Medical Treatment: Painkillers and ice/heat packs will usually be sufficient. Steroid injections and physiotherapy can also be used. If calcium deposits have built up around the tendon (calcific tendonitis), they can be removed surgically or treated with shock waves.

Prognosis: Episodes usually only last a few days but can be more persistent.

Holistic Advice: Rest the tendon during an episode. Avoid repetitive movement and exercise the affected area to strengthen the muscles around the tendon to try to avoid another episode. Warm up before exercise and cool down properly after it.

Tennis Elbow / Golfers Elbow

Definition: Inflammation of a tendon (tendonitis) at its attachment to the bone at the elbow. Tennis elbow affects the outside of the elbow and golfer's elbow affects the inner side of the elbow. Tennis elbow is referred to as lateral epicondylitis and golfer's elbow is called medial epicondylitis.

Possible Causes: Vigorous and/or repeated use of muscles in the forearm can damage the muscles and tendons. Common activities that cause overuse and hence tennis or golfer's elbow include racquet sports, sports involving throwing, swimming, and the extensive use of gardening shears. It can also be brought on by work that involves repetitive wrist action (e.g. brick laying and typing).

General Signs and Symptoms: Pain and tenderness on the outside of the elbow (tennis elbow) or the inner side (golfer's elbow). The pain may radiate down the forearm and twisting movements are often particularly painful. Repetitive wrist movements can make the pain worse. The pain may range from mild when the joint is moved, to severe pain even at rest.

Conventional Medical Treatment: Anti-inflammatory drugs can be used for the pain and, in severe cases, a corticosteroid injection may be recommended. Physiotherapy may be required to help stretch and strengthen the muscles in the forearm. Surgery can be used but only usually as a last resort.

Prognosis: In most cases the symptoms eventually clear up without treatment but tendons are slow to heal and so this may take several weeks, months or even over a year.

Holistic Advice: Try to limit the chance of damaging the tendons by warming up properly before playing sport, seek advice on sporting technique, and try to avoid movements that cause pain. Rest a painful arm as soon as possible. Ice packs may bring relief. Acupuncture claims to be effective in some cases.

Testicular Lumps (Benign)

Definition: A variety of non-cancerous lumps that may form in the testes. There are 4 main types of benign testicular lump - varicocele, hydrocele, epididymal cyst and testicular torsion.

Possible Causes: Varicocele is a collection of varicose veins in the scrotum, possibly caused by abnormalities in the veins (including weakened valves) that results in a swelling due to the accumulation of blood. Hydrocele is the accumulation of fluid in the scrotum. In adult men this may be caused by infection, inflammation or injury of the testis. An epididymal cyst is a fluid-filled swelling caused by the accumulation of skin cells and protein. A testicular torsion is caused when the testis twists on the spermatic cord within the scrotum, often interrupting the blood supply.

General Signs and Symptoms: Many lumps cause no other symptoms but are discovered by routine examinations. Others may cause a heavy sensation or pain in the scrotum or groin. Varicoceles tend not to cause any symptoms other than the swelling, develop on the left side of the scrotum and may feel like a bag of worms. Hydroceles are only evident by the swelling although the fluid may cause the scrotum to feel heavy. Epididymal cysts may become infected, in which case they can become red, painful and smelly. Testicular tortion is extremely painful and is a medical emergency. If not treated very quickly the testis may have to be removed. Sudden pain in the scrotum, groin and lower abdomen, redness and extreme tenderness of the scrotum, nausea, vomiting and a fever are typical symptoms.

Conventional Medical Treatment: Small varicoceles do not usually need to be treated and often disappear. If surgery is required the procedure is to inject the veins with a chemical that causes the veins to block. Hydroceles only tend to be treated if they are causing problems in which case the fluid is drained from the scrotum. Epididymal cysts normally remain small and do not require treatment. If they become infected corticosteroid injections can be used or they can be surgically removed. Testicular torsion is corrected by surgery.

Prognosis: With the exception of testicular torsion, benign testicular lumps do not tend to have any associated complications.

Holistic Advice: All men should be encouraged to examine their testicles regularly. Only about 4% of all testicular lumps are malignant but it is important to get a diagnosis if any testicular lump is found. Testicular cancer is one of the most easily treated cancers if detected early.

Tetanus

Definition: A bacterial infection that produces severe muscle stiffness and spasms. It is quite rare in developed countries because most people have now been immunized. Commonly called lockjaw.

Possible Causes: Caused by the Clostridium tetani bacterium, which lives in soil, dust and the manure of animals such as horses and cows. The bacteria enter the body through open wounds. Once in the body they multiply, releasing a neurotoxin. The neurotoxin is carried around the body in the bloodstream, blocking nerve impulses from the spinal cord to the muscles. There is a risk of infection when the skin is damaged by burns, and the infection can also be introduced to the body by animal bites, body piercing, tattoos, intravenous drug use etc.

General Signs and Symptoms: Symptoms develop about 10 days after infection and are typified by muscle stiffness (particularly in the face and jaws) and painful muscle spasms (particularly in the neck, throat and face). There may also be a fever, headache, rapid heart beat and hypertension. If the muscles of the throat or chest are affected it can lead to problems swallowing and breathing difficulties respectively. Spasms in the back can cause the spine to arch backwards.

Conventional Medical Treatment: Immediate treatment is required. Antitoxin injections and antibiotics may be used. Sedatives may be needed to relieve any muscle spasms.

Prognosis: If the infection is not treated immediately it can be fatal.

Holistic Advice: Keep tetanus vaccine up to date, especially if travelling or in contact with soil and manure (e.g. farming and gardening). Wash any wounds and treat them with antiseptic immediately. If not vaccinated, see a Doctor with any wounds contaminated with soil or manure or with any deep wounds.

Thrush (Vaginal)

Definition: Inflammation and irritation of the vagina and vulva caused by a fungal infection.

Possible Causes: Caused by a Candida fungal infection, most commonly the Candida albicans fungus. The Candida fungus lives naturally in the vagina without causing any problems but then conditions change and thrush is triggered. Risk factors include taking antibiotics, pregnancy, diabetes and a damaged immune system. Stress, sexual activity, tight fitting clothing, and the combined oral contraceptive pill may also be contributory triggers.

General Signs and Symptoms: Intense irritation and itching of the vagina and vulva, pain or discomfort during sex and urination, and there may be a vaginal discharge.

Conventional Medical Treatment: Anti-fungal medications can be taken either orally or inserted into the vagina. Topical creams can help soothe sore parts of the genitals.

Prognosis: Treatment is usually effective but the infection can recur.

Holistic Advice: Avoid perfumed soap or other scented products that may come into contact with the genitals, keep the genitals clean, dry and cool, wear loose fitting clothing and cotton underwear, wipe the bottom from front to back after going to the toilet, reduce stress, and avoid sex until the condition has cleared. Make sure the vagina is well lubricated before sexual intercourse, but avoid latex condoms, spermicidal creams and lubricants if they are found to cause irritation. Boost the immune system.

Tonsillitis

Definition: Inflammation of the tonsils.

Possible Causes: Can be caused by either a bacterial or, most commonly, a viral infection. Bacterial tonsillitis is likely to be caused by group A streptococcus bacteria. Viruses that affect the respiratory system, including the flu virus, are usually the ones responsible for viral tonsillitis. The Epstein-Barr virus that causes glandular fever can also cause tonsillitis.

General Signs and Symptoms: Sore throat, red, swollen tonsils, white pus-filled spots on the tonsils, pain when swallowing, fever, coughing, headache, tiredness and swollen lymph glands in the neck.

Conventional Medical Treatment: If the tonsillitis is caused by a bacterial infection antibiotics can be used. Painkillers, lozenges and throat sprays can help ease the symptoms. Tonsillectomy can be undertaken to remove the tonsils in severe or recurring cases.

Prognosis: Usually clears up on its own but in severe or recurring cases the tonsils can be removed.

Holistic Advice: Drink plenty of fluids and try to eat. Boost the immune system.

Toothache

Definition: Pain or discomfort in one or more teeth or in the gums.

Possible Causes: Toothache can be caused by many disorders of the teeth including dental decay, cavities, tooth fractures, pulpitis (inflammation of the pulp in the tooth) receding gums and abscesses. Pain may also arise from teeth that are misaligned.

General Signs and Symptoms: Pain in a tooth and/or gum that may radiate to the face, neck and ears. The pain may be worse when chewing or if the teeth are exposed to heat or cold. There may be a swelling around the affected tooth and the tooth or gums may bleed. Toothache over a period of time can affect nutrition and can be very wearing.

Conventional Medical Treatment: The treatment will depend on the cause of the pain. X-rays can help determine the extent of the problem. The tooth may be filled, capped or removed. Abscesses may be treated with antibiotics and/or drained. Root canal treatment, in which the decayed area, pulp cavity and root canals are filled, may be required if the decay invades the pulp. Painkillers can be used to help relieve the pain. Orthodontic treatments can be used to correct crowded or unevenly spaced teeth.

Prognosis: Not usually considered to be serious however, if left untreated, the infection from an abscess can spread into the bone and bloodstream causing serious complications.

Holistic Advice: Cut down on sugary foods, thoroughly brush the teeth at least twice a day, use dental floss and mouthwash to help clean between the teeth, don't smoke and visit a dentist annually for a check up.

Tuberculosis

Definition: A bacterial infection that most often affects the lungs but can affect other parts of the body. Often abbreviated to TB.

Possible Causes: Caused by the bacteria Mycobacterium tuberculosis and it is spread through the droplets of saliva dispersed by the coughs and sneezes of an infected person. In many healthy people the infection is fought off and the bacteria killed by the immune system and so the condition does not progress. In others, the TB bacteria may lie dormant and reactivate years later if the person's immunity is reduced. People with reduced immunity are at greatest risk from developing TB, e.g those with HIV, diabetes mellitus or taking immunosuppressant drugs. Other risk factors include long term lung disease, living in overcrowded conditions with poor sanitation, travelling to parts of the world where TB is more prevalent, the elderly and the very young.

General Signs and Symptoms: Initially there may be no symptoms until a cough develops and the infected person feels generally unwell. If the disease progresses the cough becomes persistent and productive, and there may be chest pain on deep inhalation, shortness of breath, fever, poor appetite, weight loss, night sweats and tiredness. If the infection spreads to other parts of the body additional symptoms are caused. Rarely the infection does not begin in the lungs, for example if unpasteurised milk is drunk from a cow infected with TB, the infection may begin in the gastrointestinal tract.

Conventional Medical Treatment: Can usually be treated effectively with a combination of oral antituberculous drugs (antibiotics) taken for about 6 months. The BCG vaccine against TB is available.

Prognosis: Left untreated it may cause long term illness and death. Some types of TB are more resistant to the drugs than others. Even treated the disease can still be fatal in those whose immunity is severely weakened.

Holistic Advice: Boost the immune system. If infected, try to prevent the spread of the disease by taking care when coughing, disposing of tissues carefully and maintaining good hand hygiene.

<u>Ulcerative Colitis</u>

Definition: Chronic intermittent inflammation and ulceration of the colon.

Possible Causes: The lining of the colon becomes inflamed, swollen and ulcerates. The ulcers can bleed and create mucus and pus. The exact cause is unknown but there may possibly be genetic and environmental links. Some believe that it may be caused by a malfunction in the immune system. Tends to develop in young adults.

General Signs and Symptoms: Diarrhoea (often containing blood and mucus), abdominal pain, tiredness, loss of appetite, weight loss, anaemia, fever, a constant need to open the bowels, and dehydration. Symptoms can range from mild to severe and the number of attacks can vary.

Conventional Medical Treatment: Mild-moderate cases can usually be successfully treated with drugs. Aminosalicylates (to reduce inflammation), steroids (if aminosalicylates are not strong enough) and immunosuppressants (also to help reduce the inflammation) can be prescribed. Surgery to remove the colon may be required. This results in a colostomy (the creation of a stoma in the abdominal wall through which faeces is passed).

Prognosis: Can usually be successfully managed but complications can arise in severe cases. Sufferers of ulcerative colitis have an increased risk of colorectal cancer. This risk increases with the length of time the condition has been present.

Holistic Advice: Keep a diary to see if any foods worsen the condition. Drink plenty of fluids. Try to reduce stress levels.

Urinary Incontinence

Definition: The complete or partial loss of voluntary control over bladder function. There are four types. 1. Stress incontinence, which is the involuntary loss of urine during exertion. 2. Urge incontinence, which is characterized by repeated episodes of involuntary loss of urine preceded by a sudden and urgent need to empty the bladder. 3. Overflow incontinence, in which there is often a blockage that prevents the bladder from emptying properly. The urine builds up and the pressure causes leaks. 4. Total incontinence, when there is no bladder control at all. We'll concentrate on stress and urge as they are the most common.

Possible Causes: Stress incontinence occurs when the pelvic floor muscles weaken to the extent that they cannot prevent urination. Pelvic muscles may weaken as a result of pregnancy, childbirth, menopause, hysterectomy, age and obesity. Urge incontinence occurs when the bladder is unstable or overactive and contracts too early, often before the bladder is full. The exact cause is unknown but it is thought to occur as a result of incorrect signals being sent between the brain and the bladder, or the irritability of the muscle in the bladder wall by infection or inflammation. Mild urinary incontinence may be triggered by some medicines (e.g. diuretics and muscle relaxants), certain drinks (e.g. alcohol, coffee (both diuretics), citrus fruit juices and drinks containing artificial sweeteners. Chronic coughing can also weaken the sphincter.

General Signs and Symptoms: The main symptom is the loss of voluntary bladder control which causes urination to take place unintentionally. Losing a small amount of urine upon activities such as coughing or sneezing is symptomatic of stress incontinence. The sudden, urgent, and usually frequent need to urinate is typical of urge incontinence. There may be only seconds between warning and urination.

Conventional Medical Treatment: The type and severity of the condition will affect the treatment. Lifestyle changes and pelvic floor exercises may help all types. For stress incontinence a number of surgical procedures are available. For urge incontinence, bladder training may help lengthen the time between feeling the need to urinate and urinating. Medication (e.g. antimuscarinics) to help relax the muscle in the bladder and surgical options are possible but not without risks.

Prognosis: Lifestyle changes may help and medical intervention can help ease the symptoms.

Holistic Advice: Reduce caffeine and alcohol intake, lose excess weight, stop smoking and ensure fluid intake is correct. This condition can be upsetting for the sufferer so remember to treat any anxiety or depression.

Varicose Veins

Definition: Swollen and enlarged veins.

Possible Causes: Varicose veins are caused by the weakening of the valves that prevent the backflow of blood in the veins. It is not fully understood why this happens but risk factors include sex (women are more likely to suffer), prolonged standing, being overweight, age, family history of the disease and pregnancy.

General Signs and Symptoms: Dark blue/purple, lumpy, bulging veins, most commonly occurring in the calves of the legs where they are visible through the skin. Some people will not experience any discomfort as a result of the varicose veins. Others may find the legs ache, throb or cramp, and the feet and ankles may swell. The skin over the affected area may also become dry, thin and itchy and occasionally leg ulcers may arise. Varicose veins can occur in other parts of the body, e.g. oesophagus, uterus, vagina, pelvis and rectum.

Conventional Medical Treatment: Treatment will only be required if the varicose veins are causing discomfort, if they are causing complications, or for cosmetic reasons. Treatments include compression stockings, sclerotherapy (in which a chemical is injected into the vein to seal it so preventing blood from entering) or surgery to remove them.

Prognosis: Varicose veins may not look nice, but they do not usually affect circulation or create any other serious health problems. Varicose veins may recur even after surgery.

Holistic Advice: Take regular exercise such as swimming and walking to keep the blood flowing in the legs. Raise the legs when resting to aid blood flow. Avoid prolonged sitting or standing and don't cross the legs when sitting. Support stockings can be beneficial, particularly to those who have to stand a lot, and avoid wearing tight clothing that restricts the blood flow at the top of the legs. Lose excess weight and stop smoking. Never massage over or below a varicose vein.